KV-194-964

Dr Richard B. Fisher received a PhD from Yale University followed by an MSc from Brunel. He came to London as founding Managing Director of a paperback book publishing house and began to write on medical subjects in 1968. He has written and presented documentaries for BBC Radio, published various articles in *The Observer Colour Magazine* and *The Guardian* and is the author of several other books including *A Dictionary of Mental Health*, *A Dictionary of Drugs* (with Dr George Christie), *A Dictionary of Body Chemistry*, a biography of Joseph Lister and *Brain Games*. In 1972, Dr Fisher became a British citizen. At the moment he is planning to drive from London to Beijing following the route used by Marco Polo in the thirteenth century.

RICHARD B. FISHER

A Dictionary of Diets, Slimming and Nutrition

PALADIN
GRAFTON BOOKS
A Division of the Collins Publishing Group

LONDON GLASGOW
TORONTO SYDNEY AUCKLAND

Paladin
Grafton Books
A Division of the Collins Publishing Group
8 Grafton Street, London W1X 3LA

A Paladin Paperback Original 1986

Copyright © Richard B. Fisher 1986

ISBN 0-586-08485-1

Printed and bound in Great Britain by
Collins, Glasgow

Set in Plantin

—

Foreword

Neither the slimming diets nor the EXERCISES* described in the *Dictionary of Diets, Slimming and Nutrition* should be undertaken unless you first obtain your doctor's approval. This rule applies especially to anyone who is pregnant or who suffers from a chronic illness.

Strident though these commands may seem, they are no more than common sense, like everything else that follows. Our object is or should be to eat for peak efficiency. Each of us knows when we eat the wrong things or simply over-eat. A 'business' lunch followed by a three-course, home-cooked dinner is more food than the average, office-bound company director needs. Anyone who has chips for lunch, cream buns with the kids' tea and dinner with their partner every day is bound to be overweight. Even a steel worker may find his body expanding if he has three square meals a day plus three pints every night.

Though you wouldn't think so from the number of new diet books that appear every year, there is no magical way to keep fit. Every diet – and most of them are sensible if occasionally just a little too intensive – depends for its effect on you. You are the one who must stick to the rules. Probably, you must eat less than you are used to eating, or at least less FAT and SUGAR.

The *Dictionary of Diets, Slimming and Nutrition* tries to help in two ways: it sets out in layman's language what you should be eating in the interests of your health, and why. It also gives you the facts on various popular diets and

---

* Words in small capitals throughout the book are the headings of entries in the *Dictionary*.

SLIMMING AIDS so that you can compare them before buying diet books or products. There is also an entry on exercise, because unless you do something with the ENERGY you eat, you cannot possibly be fit. And several entries are devoted to the much-vexed subjects of food ADDITIVES and HEALTH FOODS.

Many reference works contain a bibliography both as a source list and for further reading. Most of the data in the *Dictionary*, however, come from research papers and specialized secondary sources. For example, information on additives and food PROCESSING is taken from two books, R. J. Taylor, *Food Additives*, Wiley, 1980, and H. G. Muller and G. Tobin, *Nutrition and Food Processing*, Croom Helm, 1980, as well as several papers. A. A. Paul and D. A. T. Southgate, *The Composition of Foods* (4th edition) HMSO, 1978, is invaluable for detailed analysis of common foods. Though they are easily understood, these books were not written for a general audience. J. Yudkin, *This Nutrition Business*, Davis-Poynter, 1976, and S. Bingham, *Nutrition*, Corgi, 1978, are popular in their approach, but both are several years old, a drawback in this rapidly developing field. It is impossible to recommend anything else written for the general reader. Indeed, as you will discover in the entries themselves, I think that some of the titles mentioned contain material that is at best misleading. Were it otherwise the *Dictionary of Diets, Slimming and Nutrition* would have been less necessary.

Again, I wish to thank Dr Peter Evans, journalist and broadcaster, for his helpful comments on the manuscript.

RBF
London, 1985

A

ABSORPTION, FOOD
The process by means of which NUTRIENTS from food enter the body. Most absorption takes place in the small intestine, which is about 20 feet long, but WATER, some NUTRIENTS and other factors are also absorbed through the walls of the stomach and the large intestine including the rectum.

From the standpoint of food and nutrition, the lumen or interior of the intestines is actually outside the body. Food is of no use to us unless and until it crosses the intestinal wall. In order for nutrients to feed us, they must enter the body through the cells lining the intestines and forming their walls. In the small intestine, absorption takes place through villi, tiny projections into the intestinal lumen. The villi are covered by hair-like microvilli consisting of a single layer of cells. The villi and microvilli greatly extend the absorptive surface of the small intestine bringing millions of cells into close contact with nutrients. These cells also contain ENZYMES which complete the DIGESTIVE PROCESS.

Simple SUGARS from CARBOHYDRATES and AMINO ACIDS from PROTEINS pass through cells of the intestinal lining into capillaries in the intestinal wall. The blood transports them to the liver for processing or storage and to the muscles and other tissues. The B VITAMINS, vitamin C and many MINERALS also pass directly into the blood. LIPIDS and emulsified FATS cannot enter the capillaries, but instead are taken up by lacteals, another set of tubes in the intestinal walls. Lacteals carry lymph, a colourless fluid similar to blood plasma (blood without the blood cells), and eventually empty into blood vessels. Vitamins A, D, E and K are absorbed with fats because they are fat-soluble.

See also BILE, MALABSORPTION.

ACID
1. In common usage: sour. 2. In chemical and nutritional usage: a chemical compound consisting of hydrogen and an electrically-negative element or compound; for example,

chlorine, as in hydrochloric acid $(H+Cl-)$, or citrate as in citric acid.

Acids may be classified as strong or weak. A strong acid releases hydrogen easily. It is corrosive because the electronegative portion combines with any available electropositive substance such as IRON or copper. In food, strong acids are almost always POISON. Oxalic acid in rhubarb leaves is poisonous because there is too much of it, but the small amounts of oxalic acid in spinach or TEA are tolerated by healthy people. One strong acid, hydrochloric acid, is formed naturally by cells in the stomach wall and plays an important role in the DIGESTIVE PROCESS.

Dozens of weak acids are essential constituents of food. They include AMINO ACIDS, fatty acids (see LIPID), citric acid, nicotinic acid or VITAMIN B_3, folic acid (also a B vitamin) and the acetic acid in VINEGAR.

From the nutritional standpoint, an excessively acid diet may be as harmful as a diet lacking in vitamin C, ascorbic acid, for example. Apart from the poisonous acids, foods such as FRUIT juices can introduce too much acid into the stomach causing erosion of the mucous lining, a possible cause of ulceration (see ULCER). As with any other food constituents, food acids must be balanced by substances that act as BUFFERS.

See also, BASE.

ADDITIVE, FOOD

Substances intentionally added to food to preserve or enhance its nutritional value or to make it more palatable. Note that by this definition, the safety of food additives cannot be taken for granted. They are the subject of continuous observation and research by manufacturers, university and government institutions.

The use of food additives is nothing new. Eaten by itself, SUGAR is a food. Used to sweeten COFFEE or TEA, it becomes an additive. Probably the earliest additives were HERBS and spices. Though some are PRESERVATIVES, they were often used simply to disguise the taste of spoilage. Thus, the misuse of additives is also nothing new. What has changed is that now we expect our appointed experts to protect us against such abuses.

At the beginning of this century, there were no more than fifty additives in use, not including herbs and spices. Today, there are almost 4000. The following classes are dealt with in separate entries:

ACID	FIRMING AGENT
ANTICAKING	FLAVOUR
AGENT	HUMECTANT
ANTIOXIDANT	PRESERVATIVE
BUFFER	SEQUESTRANT
COLOUR, FOOD	STABILIZER
EMULSIFIER	SWEETENER
ENZYME	

In the UK, supervision of legislation concerning food additives is the responsibility of the Food Advisory Committee (FAC), an independent body of experts which advises the government and, in particular, the Ministry of Agriculture, Fisheries and Food on all matters relating to food. The FAC considers both the need for and the safety-in-use of each substance. On the question of safety, it is advised by the Department of Health and Social Security's Committee on Toxicity of Chemicals in Food, Consumer Products and the Environment.

In the US, regulation is under the Food and Drug Administration (FDA). In general, the FDA approves any substance as an additive that is shown to be safe in the conditions of intended use. British practice requires that in addition to safety, there should be a demonstrated need for the additive that is not met by one already permitted. Choice of additives is more restricted in the UK than in the US, and there is greater use of fewer additives.

The EEC has issued directives on the rationalization of the laws of member states regarding additives, but these directives must be given force by the respective national legislatures. The EEC has also assigned E (European) numbers to a large number of additives, and these are now used in LABELLING in the UK. However, many additives do not yet have E numbers and must be listed separately on labels.

For a list of E numbers, see Appendix II.

ALCOHOL

As ethyl alcohol or ethanol, the principal pleasure-giving constituent of BEER, SPIRITS and WINE. In excess, ethyl alcohol is a POISON. Although it is not a NUTRIENT, alcohol contains 7 CALORIES per gram, more than SUGAR, STARCH or PROTEIN and only slightly less than FAT. It is excluded from all slimming diets, at least in their early stages.

Ethyl alcohol is not normally found in the body. It is not a breakdown product of the food we eat nor of our metabolic processes (see METABOLISM). Theoretically, bacteria or YEAST in the gut could ferment partially digested food producing alcohol, but in practice it does not happen. Yeast is itself digested, and the normal bacterial inhabitants of the intestines are the wrong type. In any case, food seldom stays in the intestines long enough for FERMENTATION to take place. The body does contain some alcohols, the most familiar being CHOLESTEROL, but not ethanol.

In a drink, ethanol will be absorbed within about two hours. Prior digestion is not necessary, and ABSORPTION begins in the stomach. Effervescent drinks like champagne are absorbed more quickly. Eating or drinking MILK before a party may slow alcohol absorption, but neither provides a permanent shield. Absorption through the small intestine is not affected by the presence of other food.

Alcohol in the blood may be taken up by cells anywhere in the body. In the liver, it is slowly detoxified by the action of an ENZYME, alcohol dehydrogenase. Nerve cells are not especially avid for alcohol, but because their function is to conduct signals which alcohol inhibits, they are most noticeably affected. The higher centres of the brain which regulate self-control are the first to react followed by the senses, vision, hearing, touch, taste and smell, and muscular reaction time. When blood alcohol concentration reaches roughly 100mg per 100ml, signs of being drunk appear. About 50g of alcohol or the equivalent of three pints of bitter produce this blood concentration. In Britain, the law makes it an offence to drive with more than 80mg of alcohol per 100ml of blood, equal to about 40g of alcohol or 2½ pints for an 11-stone man.

Alcohol content may be measured as proof in the UK. A proof SPIRIT is 50 per cent alcohol by weight and 57 per cent by volume. Thus, 70 proof spirit contains 70 per cent of proof spirit by volume; therefore, $70/100 \times 57 = 40$ml of alcohol per 100ml of spirits or $40 \times 0.8 = 32$g of alcohol per 100ml. Because the ENERGY content of pure ethanol is 7 Calories per gram, the same 100ml of 70 proof spirit contains 222 Calories. There are only traces of other nutrients in spirits.

Beer and wine contain slightly larger amounts of other nutrients, but no common alcoholic beverage provides useful amounts of FAT, MINERALS, PROTEIN or VITAMINS. Alcohol itself is a CARBOHYDRATE.

Ethanol consumption in moderation may improve appetite, especially in old people. It can help people to sleep by reducing tension, and for the same reason it may calm colic. However, the warm flush that follows a drink reflects dilation of blood vessels in the skin. As an antidote to chill, alcohol may be deceptive because the more blood in the skin, the more rapidly the blood cools. Thus, alcohol can increase heat loss in people suffering from exposure. The traditional shot of brandy is appropriate only if the person is already dry and well wrapped up.

In cases of energy starvation brought on either by unusually heavy EXERCISE or by food deprivation, alcohol is definitely contraindicated. It interferes with the process by which stored sugar, GLYCOGEN, is made available as glucose, the form that cells can use to produce energy. The immediate energy that alcohol supplies cannot make up for the deficits imposed by exercise or food deprivation. In short, alcohol has its uses apart from conviviality, but they are limited.

Methyl alcohol or meths is a poison in very small quantities. It breaks down in the body to formaldehyde and formic acid. Formaldehyde quickly causes blindness.

Formic acid makes body fluids too ACID and can be fatal. The liver enzyme that breaks down methyl alcohol to formaldehyde and formic acid is alcohol dehydrogenase, the same enzyme that detoxifies ethanol. Because the enzyme reacts more efficiently with ethyl alcohol than with meths, however, spirits are a good antidote to meths poisoning. At the same time, to correct the acidosis, the patient should be given an alkali (see BASE) like sodium bicarbonate.

ALGINATE
A food ADDITIVE extracted from seaweed (genus *Laminaria*) and used as an EMULSIFIER, STABILIZER or THICKENER. Alginates contain food FIBRE. They are most commonly used in artificial cream, ice-cream, instant pudding, pie-filling of comminuted or crushed FRUIT, processed CHEESE and salad cream. Alginates may be added to antacids to protect the intestinal lining. Chemically, they are SALTS of a weak ACID, alginic acid.

ALKALI See BASE

ALLERGY, FOOD
An immunological mistake causing the body to react to non-threatening substances, in this case in food. Note that although psychological factors may make allergy worse in some people, the underlying disorder is physiological.

The immune defence system exists to protect us against potentially lethal damage by external substances and other organisms. The most obvious examples are bacteria and viruses, that is, germs, and the POISONS they synthesize, plant poisons, foreign blood and other foreign tissues. When any of these substances is brought into direct contact with body cells, the challenge produces defensive immuno-logical reactions. They are extremely complex, but we can observe them as the familiar symptoms of many different diseases: fever, sneezing, running nose, digestive disorders, inflammation, rash, headache and other pain. Incidentally, far from being uniquely human, all known organisms display immunological defences of some sort.

Unfortunately, the immune defence systems of some people go into action in response to substances that are not dangerous. This unwanted reaction is allergy, and the causative substances are allergens. Not only are some allergens like the dried grass that can cause hay fever not in themselves poisonous, but they may even contain NUTRIENTS of positive benefit. That is, they are food. No one knows why these immunological mistakes occur in one person and not in another, but a tendency to allergies seems to run in families. Not that your children will be allergic to strawberries if you are, but they are at greater risk of being allergic to something than a child of parents without allergies. Probably about 10 per cent of the population inherit a tendency to allergy.

What causes the symptoms? Immune responses are of two types, broadly speaking: natural and adaptive. Natural immune mechanisms basically exist at birth. They consist of cells which either produce chemicals designed to immobilize and destroy invaders or clean up the debris left after the battle. Some of these non-specific defence cells do both, but they are non-specific in that they are stimulated to act against any foreign invader. Most of the symptoms of immunological defence, or of allergy, reflect the activities of these non-specific natural defences. For example, throughout the body there is a class of cells called mast cells. An infection or irritation causes them to produce histamine and prostaglandins, powerful chemicals that induce inflammation, pain and other symptoms in the parts affected.

Adaptive immune responses are so called because they change and develop as the body faces new challenges. These responses also depend on cells which are of two types: T-cells and B-cells. T means thymus, a gland in the upper chest just below the neck. In infancy and early life, the thymus processes immunocompetent cells so that they acquire certain abilities, the most important being the ability to distinguish between cells that are part of the body and cells and other substances that are not. T-cells produce chemicals that enhance or suppress the reactivity of both non-specific immune defence cells and of B-cells. Thus, if an allergen appears in the body, some T-cells produce chemicals called lymphokines enhancing the reactions of other cells.

Lymphokines are also at the root of an important allergic reaction, delayed hypersensitivity. After a bee sting, for example, most people experience localized pain and swelling that reflects mobilization of natural immune defences near the sting. If you respond allergically to a bee sting, the symptoms may be much more widespread and the next time you are stung you may suffer an asthmatic attack, palpitations, even convulsions. Your doctor will no doubt prescribe pills that you should keep with you at all times in case of another sting. The machinery behind the extreme delayed hypersensitivity reaction is the T-cell lymphokines signalling the reappearance of an allergen previously experienced by the T-cell population. However, the internal signal that a new bee sting has occurred is probably the work of the second type of adaptive immune defence cell, the B-cell or, more specifically, of the antibodies B-cells produce.

B means bursa, a structure found in birds where these cells were first identified, but not in people (or other mammals). All of the higher animals have B-cells, and all of them produce antibodies. Antibodies are extraordinary PROTEIN molecules. They consist of both variable and invariable or constant regions. Like all proteins, antibodies are chains of AMINO ACIDS. Segments of the constant regions fall into five different classes, but otherwise they consist of very similar amino-acid chains. On the other hand, the variable regions end in a sequence of amino acids chemically capable of linking up with one or at most a few antigens. Thus, each antibody is specific against one or a few substances, and each B-cell produces only one antibody.

An antibody can be defined as a chemical designed to seek out and link up with an antigen. An antigen is a molecule, usually a protein, on the surface of an invader.

Allergens cause allergies because they contain antigens which stimulate one or more B-cells to produce antibodies against them. The antibodies in turn activate T-cells and enhance the action of non-specific immune defence cells.

Thus, we each possess a population of cells, B-cells, capable of synthesizing antibodies against an apparently infinite number of invasive organisms and other foreign substances. The B-cells have another remarkable feature: once they have encountered an antigen and produced an antibody against it, they subdivide forming a clone of identical cells all having learned how to produce the same antibody. In this way, the body is sensitized against the antigen. The next time it appears, the reaction against it will be significantly greater than the first time. If it is a disease-causing organism, it is hoped that the reaction will be great enough to destroy it. This is the machinery that makes vaccination an efficient method of preventing a disease. But if the antigen is house dust or egg white, and B-cells have cloned so that antibodies and the T-cells mobilize every time this antigen appears, the patient is in for some pretty uncomfortable allergic reactions.

Although a few drugs may help to reduce the impact of allergy attacks, there is no sure way of preventing them. If the allergen can be positively identified, two approaches to prevention may be effective. If it is something that can be avoided like a particular food, then the subject must avoid that food. If it is something like grass cuttings that cannot be easily avoided, then an attempt may be made to desensitize the patient. A minute dose of the allergen is injected followed by larger and larger doses. If the patient is lucky, the small dose may cause B-cells to produce antibodies against the allergen which inactivate it, though why this did not happen in the first place is completely unclear. However, some allergies do disappear unaided in time. Children are said to grow out of them, but adults do too. Possibly these changes reflect a similar but natural desensitization process.

With many allergies, the problem is that the allergen is not obvious. Foods, for example, seldom consist of single chemicals. Thus, MILK is one of the most common food allergens. It can be removed from the diet without serious effects, but if the actual allergen is some constituent of milk, perhaps a small non-protein molecule such as lime which can turn up in traces in many foods, avoiding the allergen is that much more difficult.

Milk, EGGS, wheat, FISH, shellfish, bananas, strawberries, tomatoes, pork (and sometimes other MEAT), NUTS and chocolate are thought to be the most common causes of food allergies. Note that adverse reactions such as migraine to chocolate, CHEESE or red WINE are probably not allergic but rather the effect of a chemical, tyramine, contained in these foods. On the other hand, there is now evidence that in some people, migraine is caused by food allergy. The allergens certainly include milk, wheat products and eggs. COELIAC DISEASE and possibly IRRITABLE BOWEL SYNDROME are also associated with allergic reactions to foods.

Whether or not there is a more generalized condition identifiable as food allergy is highly controversial. One test published in 1983 showed by rigid scientific experimental techniques that of twenty-three adult patients who attributed a wide variety of symptoms to food allergy, hypersensitivity (that is, allergic reactions that could be identified in products of the immune system) occurred in only four. One of the four was allergic to fish, one to peas and beans and a third to oranges and tomatoes. None of these four patients showed any psychological symptoms, but psychiatric disorders were common among the remaining nineteen. None of the twenty-three patients had come to their doctors with psychiatric symptoms as such, however. Six of the nineteen patients in whom food allergy could not be confirmed first claimed that their symptoms were caused by food allergies after reading the book, *Not All in the Mind* (R. Mackarness, 1976) which argues that food allergies are more common than medical authorities believe. This fact suggests that their symptoms were of psychological origin and were identified as food allergy by these patients because they had read the book. Only the repetition of tests such as this one can indicate whether or not food allergy is more common than it now seems to be.

AMINO ACID

A small molecule that links up with other amino acids to form PROTEIN. Proteins are formed from amino acids produced in the body as well as those in food. Amino acids are also the building blocks of several HORMONES. Two or possibly three also act as chemical signals between nerve cells in the brain.

About twenty of these important molecules occur in all living organisms. In addition to the carbon, hydrogen and oxygen that constitute the bulk of all organic molecules, amino acids contain nitrogen. Three of them also contain SULPHUR. Although they are synthesized in all plants and animals, only a limited number of plants and many bacteria are capable of extracting nitrogen from the environment and fixing it in the organic molecule. All higher animals including humans and most plants must obtain their nitrogen already made up into amino acids. However, given an adequate supply of amino acids, even these organisms can convert one to another to meet their needs.

There are exceptions. For example, our bodies are capable of synthesizing only small amounts of eight amino acids, too little to meet our needs. These eight are:

Isoleucine	Phenylalanine
Leucine	Threonine
Lysine	Tryptophan
Methionine	Valine

Two more amino acids, cystine and tyrosine, are sometimes added to the list because if they are present in the diet, the need for dietary methionine and PHENYLALANINE, respectively, is reduced. These ten are called essential amino acids and must be obtained from the digestive breakdown of proteins in food. But see also, SOYA BEAN.

Animal protein from CHEESE, EGGS, FISH, MEAT or MILK provide more of the essential amino acids than VEGETABLE proteins. Thus, polished rice has very little lysine. Lysine and methionine are low in potatoes and wheat. Indeed, despite the fact that they represent the richest single source of protein, SOYA BEANS lack methionine. For this reason, it is desirable to eat some animal products or YEAST with vegetables (see VEGAN, VEGETARIAN).

If the diet lacks adequate essential amino acids, deficiency diseases develop and can be serious. For example, children fed on little beside cassava (see TAPIOCA) develop KWASHI-ORKOR. Too little tryptophan can be a contributory factor in pellagra, the disease caused by deficiency of VITAMIN B_3, niacin. At least one disease, phenylketonuria, is caused by too much of the essential amino acid, phenylalanine. It is an inherited disorder. The cells of affected individuals fail to produce an ENZYME that breaks down phenylalanine. Fortunately, infants at risk can be screened before birth and their diets adjusted to reduce phenylalanine intake.

Amino acids are weak ACIDS. They cause proteins to act as electrochemically negative compounds. Many more than twenty exist in nature, and a handful also play roles in our bodies though they are not incorporated into proteins.

ANOREXIA

Loss of appetite, lack of a desire to eat.

Anorexia can be a symptom of many diseases ranging from colds and flu to digestive disorders. It may also reflect emotional problems, for example, worry, fear or anger, and mental diseases such as anxiety and depression.

The physiological reasons for anorexia are not so easy to explain. Nerve cells regulating both the desire to eat and feelings of satiation exist in a part of the brain called the hypothalamus. It is not known if anorexia in humans involves these nerves, but in animal experiments it is possible to create anorexia even after a period of starvation by stimulating the relevant brain region.

See also ANOREXIA NERVOSA, BULIMIA.

ANOREXIA NERVOSA

A mental disorder characterized by refusal to eat, need for constant exercise and insomnia. Most patients are women aged between eighteen and twenty-five, but patients may be both younger and older. In rare cases, the patients are young men.

Though psychotherapy and careful nursing eventually restore most patients to normal physical health and weight, after-effects such as neurosis and sexual frigidity are common. About one in ten patients dies from anorexia nervosa, a shockingly high mortality for a mental disorder.

Because dieting is so common, especially among young women, the onset of symptoms may go unnoticed. Only when the patient loses three or four stone do parents or friends become suspicious. By that time, the patient's breasts will have shrunk and her periods stopped. Indeed, in many patients, the disease may be brought on by anxiety about sexual roles or relationships. Some women, for example, develop anorexia nervosa after they become engaged. In others, the triggering events, if they can be discovered at all, are more common like the death of a parent or career anxiety.

Attempts to force feed the patient are no longer made because she almost invariably vomits unwanted food. When the weight loss is severe, the patient must be hospitalized to control the amount of EXERCISE she takes and to reduce the dangers from infections arising from the weakening of her immune defences (see ALLERGY, FOOD).

See also BULIMIA.

ANTICAKING AGENT

A food ADDITIVE intended to keep the product dry. These agents are added in minute quantities to substances that moisture makes less usable either because, like flour, they become lumpy and slowly turn to paste, or because, like dried foods, they deteriorate in the presence of WATER.

Two chemical types of anticaking agent are permitted in the UK: compounds that form hydrates in the presence of water and those that adsorb or collect water without becoming damp themselves. Those that form hydrates include sodium pyrophosphate. The adsorbents include CALCIUM and bone phosphate, magnesium carbonate and several silicates.

Anticaking agents differ in their strength and their length of life. They also impart different degrees of alkalinity (see BASE) to foods.

ANTIOXIDANT

A food ADDITIVE used primarily to prevent FATS from turning rancid and to protect VITAMINS and other factors in stored foods and drinks that deteriorate in the presence of oxygen. Foods in which antioxidants are used include butter and lard, fatty CHEESES, baby foods, stored fresh FRUIT, MEAT, bakery products and BEER.

Chemically, antioxidants prevent OXIDATION of unsaturated fatty acids (see LIPID). In the presence of oxygen, these compounds break down into smaller carbon-based molecules, aldehydes and KETONES. Some produce a FLAVOUR taint when they are present in less than one part per million. Such breakdown products may become toxic, but their taste is so obnoxious that food is unlikely to be eaten long before it is dangerous.

In addition to protecting the flavour of food, antioxidants assure the supply of an essential NUTRIENT, linoleic acid. Linoleic acid is a fatty acid that our body cells cannot synthesize. It must be supplied in food like a vitamin. It is required for biosynthesis of cell membranes and a HORMONE, prostaglandin.

Antioxidants work because they combine with intermediate substances in the breakdown of unsaturated fatty acids. The intermediates are called free radicals, highly unstable compounds which the antioxidant stabilizes.

In the UK, antioxidants include both natural and synthetic substances. The natural antioxidants are tocopherol, a derivative of vitamin E, and ascorbates. Ascorbates are related to ascorbic acid, vitamin C, which is itself an antioxidant. The most widely used synthetic antioxidants are BHT (butylated hydroxytoluene), BTA (butylated hydroxyanisole) and three compounds called gallates. Synthetic antioxidants are not permitted in baby foods, but tocopherol is commonly used. Ascorbic acid or the ascorbates are preferred for moist foods.

APISATE ®
A SLIMMING AID available on prescription only.

Apisate is derived from amphetamine, an addictive drug no longer used for weight control. Apisate may have some of the same side-effects as amphetamine: agitation, insomnia, rapid heart beat, digestive upset, dizziness, tremor, restlessness, headache, chills, psychotic episodes and, indeed, addiction. It will not usually be prescribed for people with heart disease, diabetes or personality disturbances. Patients with glaucoma or THYROID disorders should never use Apisate. Because tolerance to the drug develops, moreover, slimmers may find that it becomes ineffective.

The common chemical name of Apisate is diethylpropion hydrochloride. See also *Tenuate*.

ASPARTAME
An artificial SWEETENER, trade name Canderal.

Aspartame is 140 to 180 times as sweet as ordinary white SUGAR (sucrose) but it contains almost no CALORIES. As of September 1983, it has been approved in the UK for domestic use and as a commercial ADDITIVE. Chemically, it is an ester or combination of a weak ACID, aspartic acid, and the AMINO ACID, PHENYLALANINE. Because aspartame releases phenylalanine when it is broken down by the body, people with phenylketonuria are recommended not to use it or food or SOFT DRINKS containing it.

See also SACCHARIN.

ATKINS DIET
A high PROTEIN, high FAT diet that replaces CALORIE counting with a urine-testing kit. It was invented by an American doctor, Robert C. Atkins.

The Atkins regimen, set forth in his book *Diet Revolution* (1974), permits unlimited food intake of anything except CARBOHYDRATE. This means no ALCOHOL, BREAD, FRUIT, potatoes, pasta, pastries, SUGAR or other sweets. Permitted foods include MEAT, FISH, POULTRY and CHEESE, all of which contain some carbohydrates, along with salads, clear SOUPS and lemon TEA. In the later stages of the diet, fruit and some bread may be added, but sugar and sweets are banned for ever.

Atkins specifically instructs his readers to consult their doctors before beginning his diet, as do many other popular diet writers. Nevertheless, the Atkins diet has aroused opposition from the American Medical Association. By removing carbohydrate, the quickest source of ENERGY, the body is forced to fall back on fat and protein, in that order. Very much the same thing happens in DIABETES. In effect, the Atkins diet creates a diabetes-like environment in the body. Unable to obtain sugar, cells convert fat to sugar. Of course this means that weight is lost, but in the process of fat conversion, KETONES are produced leading to the condition called ketosis. For the Atkins diet to work, dieters are required to make themselves more or less permanently ketotic. To be sure that they have attained this abnormal and potentially hazardous condition, Dr Atkins prescribes urine testing every five days. He recommends a chemically-prepared strip of paper that turns purple in the presence of ketones. Called 'Ketostix' in the US, the strips are not regularly available from dispensing chemists in the UK. In the first week, the strip must turn a dark purple colour. If it does not, salads are to be removed from the diet. In later stages, the dieter may eat a little more carbohydrate providing that the paper strips display at least a lavender hue at all times. If they stay pink, the dieter is expected to return to an earlier, more rigid stage of the diet. Pink means that the urine is relatively non-acid, or more normal. The dieter is also expected to keep a food diary so that if the urine test becomes pink, as it were, it will be clear what has done the mischief. In his books, Dr Atkins provides guidance to the carbohydrate content of common foods.

There is no doubt that a diet free of sugar and most STARCH will lead to weight loss even if the Calorie content is high. Not only does the body eat up its own fat and possibly its protein to obtain energy, but it also expends energy in the process. Of course, a long-term shift in eating patterns combined with the urine test may help. As Dr Atkins recognizes, 'the main change that has to be made is in your head' if you want to lose weight. Whether the intentional induction of an abnormal physical state is a sensible means for achieving a desirable end is at best controversial.

AYDS ®

Tablets used to reduce appetite. Ayds is a food, not a drug, and may be bought without prescription as a SLIMMING AID. AYDS may reduce appetite like any other snack taken before a meal, but unlike the usual snack, the product contains a good selection of nutrients and very few CALORIES.

It consists of cubes, one or two of which are to be taken twenty minutes before each meal. Each cube has 23 Calories and contains SUGAR, sweetened condensed skimmed MILK and various other less important ingredients. In addition to CARBOHYDRATES, FAT and PROTEIN, Ayds consist of CALCIUM, IRON and PHOSPHORUS and VITAMINS A, B_1, B_2 and B_3.

See also BRAN-SLIM.

B

BASE

A substance which has an opposite effect to that of an ACID on food and body fluids. Although acid also means sour, bases are not sweet, nor are SWEETENERS basic. However, many bases are also alkalis.

In chemical terms, a base is any compound that combines with an acid to produce a SALT and WATER. It may also be defined technically as a substance which accepts protons or gives up hydroxyl (OH) ions in water and, for these reasons, raises the pH of the mixture above 7. It is this last quality which makes alkalis basic.

Alkalis are substances such as SODIUM or POTASSIUM

hydroxide. These combinations of a light metal and water are common constituents of organic compounds including foods. They may also be used as ADDITIVES. Perhaps the most familiar base in foods is sodium bicarbonate, but it is not an alkali. Other basic additives include sodium, potassium and magnesium carbonates. They are all used as BUFFERS to counteract acidity.

See also SEQUESTRANT.

BEER

An alcoholic drink obtained by fermenting CEREALS.

British beers were originally FERMENTATIONS of any available cereal. In Europe and America today, barley is the common cereal used to make beer. Beer, especially stout, is often part of post-operative or post-illness diets because it enhances the patient's sense of well-being, and because it also contributes ENERGY in the form of ALCOHOL and CARBOHYDRATES.

The barley is first malted by allowing it to sprout so that ENZYMES will convert the STARCH in the seed to a SUGAR, maltose, and other carbohydrates. WATER, hops and more sugar are added to the malt before infusion of YEAST, the organism which performs the fermentation process. Beer and ale are produced by one kind of yeast, and lager by another which ferments from the bottom of the vat, increasing the effervescence. Hops flavour beer and preserve it by inhibiting bacterial growth.

Beer contains 2 per cent to 4 per cent alcohol by weight. The following table compares the alcohol content and caloric value of various types of beer with cider, SPIRITS and WINE.

	Alcohol		Calories	
	g/100ml	g/pint	per 100ml	per pint
Bitter	3.1	17.4	32	177
Pale ale (bottled)	3.3	19	32	184
Stout (bottled)	2.9	16.3	37	212
Strong ale	6.6	37.7	72	414
Brown ale (bottled)	2.2	12.7	28	159

| | Alcohol | | Calories | |
	g/100ml	g/pint	per 100ml	per pint
and for comparison				
Cider (dry)	3.8	31.5	36	209
Red wine (approx)	9.5		68	
Spirits (70 proof)	31.7		222	

Stouts and strong ales are more caloric than cider and wine, but all other beers have fewer Calories than other alcoholic drinks and many SOFT DRINKS. Beer contains most of the B VITAMINS, the exception being B_1. It has no other vitamins and only traces of MINERALS and PROTEIN.

BEVERLY HILLS DIET

A high CARBOHYDRATE, low PROTEIN diet. CALORIE reduction is achieved by restricting food intake to FRUIT and Calorie-free beverages, COFFEE, TEA or uncarbonated WATER, during the first ten days. In order to reduce SALT intake and keep body water to a minimum, diet drinks, mineral water and any other drinks containing salt are excluded. The diet is spelled out in *The Beverly Hills Diet* (1983) by a resident of Beverly Hills, California, Judy Mazel.

The diet is presented as a discovery based on nutritional and physiological facts. Although the basic nutritional assumptions are sound enough, and very old hat, much of the data offered by way of explanation are misleading, confused or dead wrong. For example, it is not true that glucose is absorbed through the roof of the mouth, nor does the scientific literature provide references to an ENZYME called 'bromaline' which the author claims to have found in pineapple and strawberries. If she means bromelain, it is a TENDERIZER applied to MEAT before cooking and, like any other enzyme, would be destroyed during the DIGESTIVE PROCESS.

According to the author, proteins stay in the stomach for several hours, preventing the passage of carbohydrates and fruit or their waste products. In fact, it is FATS that remain longest in the stomach, but it is doubtful that they delay more than marginally the clearance of other NUTRIENTS. Finally, the author seems to believe that these 'blocked wastes' turn to ALCOHOL in the stomach, a conversion that might delight many of us if only it occurred.

Foods are assigned to the usual nutritional categories, carbohydrates, fats, proteins, to which Ms Mazel has added legumes (see PULSES) for some curious reason. The criteria governing the assignment of foods to these categories are unclear, however. For example, dairy protein is assigned to protein. Yet CHEESE, MILK, ice-cream and cheesecake contain far more fat than protein, and in the latter two, carbohydrates also outweigh protein. The reader learns that fruit (classified as carbohydrate) is digested in the mouth (not true) and fats in the stomach (also not true).

In any case, the dieter becomes a Conscious Combiner. After the first ten days on fruit only, non-fruit carbohydrates are all right, providing they are eaten before but not after protein. Fruits combine with anything, in the sense that they do not block wastes, again with the proviso that you don't eat protein afterwards.

The selling point of *The Beverly Hills Diet* is precisely that after the first weeks, you can eat as you please. There are two 'buts'. First, you must follow the rules of Conscious Combining. Second, after every food binge, you must eat nothing but fruit again for up to three days. Thus, without explaining why, the author proposes that the dieter counteract over-eating by near starvation. She capitalizes on the tendency among dieters to feel guilt after excessive eating and tries to exploit that guilt.

However nonsensical its 'science', the diet will work. In Britain, it may be a little hard to find the requisite quantity of papayas and mangoes, this being a California diet, but eating nothing but fruit for a few days will almost certainly produce a loss of weight. The diet encourages you to eat as much fruit as you want, but note that fresh pineapple, one of the principal ingredients of the diet, contains just over 200 Calories per pound. If we estimate that pineapples weigh about a pound each, the dieter will have to eat eight to ten pineapples a day just to keep level.

The relative absence of FIBRE and bulk may cause temporary constipation, but the other nutritional deficits in such a diet, deficits of protein and most VITAMINS (the exception is vitamin C), are unlikely to harm a normal adult for up to ten days. Diabetics, people with blood pressure problems and pregnant women should not attempt the Beverly Hills Diet. In any case, both the author and the publisher warn readers to seek a doctor's advice before dieting if they have any health problems at all.

BILE

The secretion of the liver which is essential for FAT digestion (see DIGESTIVE PROCESS).

Unlike CARBOHYDRATE, MINERALS and PROTEIN, all of which dissolve in WATER in the forms found in food, fats are insoluble. Without bile, they are poorly absorbed through the cells of the intestinal wall.

Bile is a mixture of compounds, but from the standpoint of fat digestion, the active ingredients are bile SALTS, glycocholate and taurocholate. Each consists of molecules with two ends, one of which is soluble in water whereas the other is not (see also LIPID). In the watery environment within the small intestine, bile salt molecules tend to arrange themselves into tiny balls called micelles. The outside is water-soluble and the inside, water-repellent. Fat molecules from foods which have been broken down in the stomach are entrapped by these molecular cages. The minute, fat-containing micelles pass through cell walls in the intestinal villi and eventually enter the circulation.

Bile assists the ABSORPTION of fatty substances such as cholesterol and the fat-soluble VITAMINS, A, D, E and K. Its alkalinity (see BASE) counteracts the effects of stomach acids and probably enhances the absorption of other NUTRIENTS. Bile also acts as a vehicle for removal of some fat wastes in the faeces.

Bile is normally a viscous fluid, brownish-yellow to green in colour. It is secreted by the liver and collected and stored in the gall bladder. Fat in the duodenum, the upper part of the small intestine, stimulates a HORMONE,

cholecystokinin, which causes the gall bladder to contract
and discharge bile. If disease or injury blocks the ducts so
that bile salts build up in the blood, the skin and eyes
become yellow. This condition is called jaundice. It may
reflect other disorders, however, and is never to be taken
lightly.

BORAGE

A common garden HERB (*Borago officianalis*) sometimes
confused with bugloss (*Lycopsis larvensis*) or *langue de boeuf*.

Borage grows to a foot or so in height with long, rough
green leaves, a reddish stalk and, in June or July, small
yellow flowers. The seeds and leaves are believed to contain
substances that add generally to one's sense of well-being.
They are best used as juice or as a syrup boiled from the
plant. Borage may serve as a mild seasoning, and is
sometimes sprinkled on salads. The flowers can be made
into jam or candied.

BRAN

The inner husk of the wheat grain minus the outer protective sheath. It is a tough, fibrous substance providing bulk
and roughage which may contribute both to the sense of
satiation and increase the speed of movement of NUTRIENTS
and wastes through the intestines. In the latter role, bran
may serve as a laxative (see also EPSOM SALTS). Its FIBRE is
neither digested nor absorbed.

Bran represents about 13 per cent of the whole grain. It
consists of CARBOHYDRATES, mostly indigestible CELLULOSE
(63 per cent), PROTEIN (17 per cent), WATER (12 per cent),
MINERALS (5 per cent), mainly MAGNESIUM, PHOSPHORUS
and POTASSIUM and fat (3 per cent). Six teaspoons of bran,
about 20g (0.7oz), taken with FRUIT or MILK or in SOUP or
YOGHURT each day will certainly relieve constipation. Five
or six slices of wholemeal BREAD give about the same
amount of FIBRE.

Bran can be bought as a raw product or as 'all bran'

breakfast CEREALS. It should be stored in airtight containers in a dry place.

See also BRAN-SLIM.

BRAN-SLIM ®
Tablets to be used as a SLIMMING AID. Their function is to reduce the appetite. Bran-Slim is a food and may be purchased without a prescription.

The manufacturer recommends one or two tablets ten minutes before a meal and between meals instead of snacks. They are made from wheat BRAN, SUGAR, gum arabic (a non-digestible CARBOHYDRATE), STARCH, HONEY and several minor ingredients. The package contains sixty tablets each of which consists of PROTEIN (0.11g), FAT (0.08g) and carbohydrate (1.04g). Each tablet has 6 CALORIES.

You should not eat Bran-Slim if you have abdominal pain, nausea, vomiting or other symptoms of appendicitis.

See also AYDS.

BREAD
A food composed of dough made from flour, WATER and YEAST which has been fermented and then baked. This entry will describe:

1. Breadmaking
2. Types of bread
3. Constituents
4. Additives
5. Storage and use

1. Breadmaking. A review of the process will introduce some of the special terms associated with this highly nutritious food. The grains of wheat or other cereals must first be milled into flour. In Britain, it was only after repeal of the Corn Laws in 1846 opened the way to hard wheats from abroad that it became possible to eliminate both BRAN and wheat germ to make white flour with the loss of important NUTRIENTS and FIBRE.

It was customary to age flour for three or four weeks

before use so that a mild oxidative process (see OXIDATION) could cause the principal wheat PROTEIN, GLUTEN, to toughen and become more elastic, increasing the loaf size. In large-scale commercial baking, however, ageing takes too long to be economically viable. It has been replaced by ripening. Improvers are added to the flour (see **Additives**, below) which produce the effects of ageing within a few hours.

The aged flour is mixed with water and kneaded to stretch the gluten and begin the process of aeration that traps gases in the dough and subsequently raises it. Yeast or some other raising agent such as bicarbonate of soda (see soda bread, below) is added to the dough shortly before baking. Yeast causes FERMENTATION which produces more gases. The fermentation process also creates small amounts of ALCOHOL, but this is driven off during baking.

The heat of baking causes tiny amounts of natural SUGAR at the surface of the loaf to caramelize, colouring the crust. The yeast as well as small amounts of added SALT impart FLAVOUR. Crusty loaves are baked more slowly at lower temperatures than slicing loaves with softer crusts.

2. Types of bread. The three main types are white, brown and wholemeal. In addition, many shops sell loaves called granary, wheat germ, soda, rye, high protein and gluten-free breads.

Wholemeal bread may also be called wholewheat. The law requires that either name must designate a bread made from water, yeast and wholemeal flour; that is, flour containing all parts of the wheat grain. Wholemeal is 100 per cent extraction flour. In other words, a pound of wheat produces a pound of flour. Obviously, wholemeal flour contains all nutrients and fibre in the wheat from which it is made.

Despite its nutritional advantages, however, the wholeness of wholewheat is not an unmixed blessing. A substance in wheat called phytic acid combines with the principal MINERALS (see **Constituents**, below) forming indigestible salts. That is, most of the minerals are lost as wastes.

Traditional methods of ageing flour (see above) gave ENZYMES in the wheat an opportunity to break down phytic acid, but the new ripening methods leave it untouched. White flour, on the other hand, loses almost all of its phytic acid during milling. Before this was appreciated, during World War II, CALCIUM in the form of chalk was added to all flour except wholemeal because it was believed that wholemeal provided adequate amounts of this important mineral. The wartime regulation remains in force because calcium may also help to prevent heart disease. Therefore, white and brown flour have four to six times the available calcium content of wholemeal.

Only three ADDITIVES are permitted in wholemeal flour. Two are improvers, ascorbic acid (VITAMIN C) and an AMINO ACID, L-cysteine hydrochloride. The third is soya flour (see SOYA BEAN). The use of British-grown soft-wheat flours (see CEREAL) has led to the addition of small amounts of soya flour to all types of wheat flour. Soya increases the protein content enhancing the size and elasticity of the loaf. It also adds more of three essential amino acids: lysine, leucine and isoleucine.

Wholemeal bread contains more nutrients and fibre than any other type (see Table, below), though with the possible exception of the fibre, the actual benefits to health remain controversial. Wholemeal bread is drier to the taste than white or brown, and people have a tendency to use more butter or other spreads with it. The effect of phytic acid, moreover, has been noted above.

White bread is made with flour from which the bran and wheat germ have been removed leaving a creamy white residue. It amounts to about 72 per cent of the original wheat by weight. Most of the B vitamins, vitamin E, minerals and fibre are removed in the process. Since 1945, the law has required that suitable amounts of IRON and vitamins B_1 (thiamin) and B_3 (niacin) are added back to white flour. Calcium is also added, and a number of other additives are permitted. They are improvers, bleaching agents, PRESERVATIVES and STABILIZERS. Soya flour may also be used.

Brown bread is made from flour produced either at an intermediate stage in the milling process or by adding bran back to white flour. Brown flour has a legal minimum fibre content of 0.6 per cent. White flour contains 0.2 per cent fibre and wholemeal, approximately 2 per cent or ten times as much as white. The law regulating additives is the same as for white flour.

Granary bread is brown bread to which malted flour (see MALT) has been added along with whole grains of wheat or other cereals. Its nutritional content is about the same as brown bread. The name is promotional rather than descriptive.

Wheat germ bread is now usually identified as brown or wholemeal, 'with added wheat germ'. At least 10 per cent of the germ must be added back to the flour which is usually brown. The law regulating additives is the same as for white flour.

Soda bread is leavened with bicarbonate of soda or another raising agent but not yeast. Non-yeast raising agents tend to be alkaline (see BASE), and alkalinity destroys vitamin B_1. Therefore, soda bread contains less B_1 than yeast leavened bread. It is made from brown, white or wholemeal flour.

Rye bread contains 20 to 60 per cent rye flour. Citric acid may be used to increase sourness, and caramel, to darken the loaf.

High-protein bread is also called starch-reduced. It contains added gluten or soya flour. Whereas ordinary bread has about 13 per cent protein, this type has between 16 and 32 per cent. Automatically, the proportion of STARCH is lowered, but high-protein bread contains about the same CALORIES as ordinary loaves because protein and CARBOHYDRATE (in the form of starch) have about the same caloric value. High-protein bread is no less fattening than ordinary bread. Permitted additives depend on the type of flour used.

Gluten-free bread is made with flour from which the gluten has been removed. It is often prescribed for people suffering from COELIAC DISEASE, phenylketonuria (see PHE-NYLALANINE) and some kidney diseases. Because the texture of a bread lacking protein entirely would be like hard biscuits, gluten is replaced by milk or egg protein.

Salt-free bread may be prescribed for people on very low-salt diets, especially patients with serious heart disease. Salt-free bread tends to stale more quickly and to have less taste.

3. Constituents.

The table compares some nutrients and other constituents in the major types of bread:

1 thin slice, about 25g	Whole-meal	White	Brown	Granary	Wheat-germ*	Standard adult daily requirement
Fibre (g)	2.1	0.7	1.3	1.3	1.15	about 25
Calories	54	58	56	57	57	2200–2600
Protein (g)	2.2	2.0	2.2	2.2	2.4	55–65
Fat (g)	0.7	0.4	0.5	0.5	0.5	
Carbohydrate (g)	10.4	12.4	11.2	11.2	11.3	
Minerals:						
Calcium† (mg)	6	25	25	25	37.5	500
Iron** (mg)	0.6	0.4	0.4	0.6	1.0	10
Magnesium (mg)	23.25	6.5	18.75	18.75	15	
Phosphorus† (mg)	57.5	24.25	47.5	47.5	47.5	
Potassium (mg)	55	25	52.5	52.5	52.5	
Sodium (mg)	125	125	137.5	137.5	145	
Others	Traces, but more in wholemeal					
Vitamins:						
A	None					750 microg
C	None					30 mg
D	None					2.5 microg
E	Traces, but slightly more in wholemeal					
B_1** (mg)	0.065	0.045	0.0575	0.0575	0.13	0.9–1.1
B_2 (mg)	0.02	0.009	0.015	0.015	0.025	1.3–1.7
B_3** (mg)	1.4	0.75	1.18	1.18	1.48	15–18 microg
B_6	Traces, but more in wholemeal					
Folic acid†† (mg)	9.75	6.75	9	9	5	
B_{12}	None					

* Hovis.

† Wholemeal flour has more calcium than the refined wheat flours, but it is not usuallly available for absorption because of the phytic acid (see **Types of bread**, above). Magnesium and iron are similarly affected. Most of the phosphorus in wholemeal flour is in the form of phytic acid.

** Added to white flour by law. Vitamin B_3 is added as a combination of the vitamin plus its precursor, tryptophan, an amino acid. Wheat normally contains both.

†† Folic acid is also a total figure, but for chemical reasons, not all the vitamin may be absorbed.

4. Additives. Eight different kinds are permitted:

i) Nutrients (none permitted in wholemeal):
Calcium
Iron
Vitamins B_1 and B_3

ii) Improvers (see **Breadmaking,** above):
Vitamin C, ascorbic acid (also permitted in wholemeal)
L-cysteine hydrochloride (also permitted in wholemeal)
Potassium bromate
Potassium persulphate (used in Scotland and northern England)
Azodicarbonaminde
Chlorine dioxide

iii) Bleaches (not permitted in wholemeal):
Benzoyl chloride (destroys vitamin E)

iv) Yeast-stimulating compounds:
Ammonium chloride
Calcium sulphate

v) Enzymes (see **Breadmaking,** above):
Malt flour
Soya flour
Amylases (break down starch)
Proteinases (break down protein)
Lipoxidases (break down fats)

vi) Colour: Caramel (not used in white)

vii) Emulsifiers:
LECITHIN
Mono- and diglycerides (see LIPID)
Stearyl tartrate
Sodium or calcium stearyl-2-lactylate

viii) Preservatives: Propionic acid (used only in flour)

5. Storage and use. As the standard of living has risen, bread consumption has declined. Diet has become more varied. Between 1956 and 1973 in Britain, average consumption per person per day declined from five and a half to four large slices. Bread has unjustifiably acquired the attribute 'fattening', like that other staple food, potatoes. Bread contains very little fat. Its Calorie content is roughly analogous to eggs: one slice of bread equals one egg. The spreads used on bread are often fattening, but bread itself is much maligned. The nutrients it contains, moreover, make it an excellent buy.

Despite additives, bread will stale. The chemical changes that take place in the starch cannot be permanently prevented. Incidentally, the same changes cause puddings and sauces to thicken and set. Staling can be delayed by careful storage in airtight bags, but beware of the mould that may then appear. Heating stale bread in the oven will sometimes restore a degree of freshness.

Toasting destroys up to 30 per cent of vitamin B_1, more in thin than thick slices. Toasting dries out the bread and browns the surface by carmelization of sugars. It does not reduce the Calorie content unless the surface is burnt so that ash replaces some of the nutrients, but most people find burnt toast unpalatable.

See also CEREAL.

BUFFER

1. A substance which maintains the acid-BASE balance of a solution at approximately neutral. 2. A food ADDITIVE used in the baking and SOFT DRINKS industries to reduce acidity (see ACID). In baking, the buffer is needed because carbon dioxide introduced to make batter porous forms acidic compounds. In soft drinks, acidic substances may be introduced as flavouring.

All permitted buffers occur naturally in human tissue as well as in food. They are either weak acids or their SALTS:

Acid	Salt
acetic acid	acetate
citric acid	citrate
fumaric acid	fumarate
lactic acid	lactate
malic acid	malate
phosphoric acid	pyrophosphate, orthophosphate

Acid	Salt
pyruvic acid	pyruvate
succinic acid	succinate
tartaric acid	tartrate

All of these substances are found naturally in the body. They act as buffers because, in solution, they dissociate only partially into positive hydrogen ions and negative ions. In the presence of a strong base, the negative ions are neutralized whereupon the buffer dissociates further to supply more negative ions, maintaining the original balance. Salts dissociate in an analogous way, and their negative ions combine with the hydrogen ions in stronger acids or in WATER. Again, the formation of the weak acid encourages the buffer salt to dissociate further, restoring the balance.

BULIMIA NERVOSA
A chronic phase of ANOREXIA NERVOSA during which the patient goes through bouts of gross over-eating followed by self-induced vomiting or purging. Bulimia means insatiable eating. Yet it is also characteristic of this condition, like anorexia nervosa, that the patient has a horror of getting fat.

The patient diets persistently, trying to avoid all fattening foods. With frequencies ranging from once a week to several times a day, she will be compelled to eat a huge snack, a whole loaf of BREAD or several chocolate bars. As much as three kilograms of highly-caloric food will be eaten quickly. Immediately the craving is satisfied, but usually furtively, the patient sticks her finger or a toothbrush handle down her throat until she vomits. Many learn to induce vomiting at will. They may also use a purgative.

Bulimic patients are seldom as thin as anorexic patients, and they often continue to menstruate. Many have calluses where the teeth rub the skin on the back of the hand that is used to induce vomiting. Patients are totally preoccupied with food and frequently depressed. In fact, the risk of suicide is greater than during anorexia nervosa.

One theory suggests that bulimia is a response by nerve

cells in the brain to years of underweight brought on by anorexia. The only treatment is hospital care, but the outlook is not hopeful.

BURDOCK
(*Arctium lappa*) A wild grass and garden weed. It has a pleasant taste, especially when prepared as an infusion in WATER. Some believe it is a tonic and blood purifier.

C

CAFFEINE
A drug found in cocoa, COFFEE and TEA. Caffeine is a stimulant. It excites nerve cells in the brain, tending to increase wakefulness and urine output and to speed up heartbeat, among other effects. Chemically, it is an alkaloid, a basic (see BASE) compound derived from a plant which contains some nitrogen as well as carbon and hydrogen. Morphine and nicotine are also alkaloids.

CALCIUM
A MINERAL needed by the body to make bones, teeth and nails. Nervous and muscular activity and blood clotting also require calcium.

In Britain, the recommended daily adult intake of this important NUTRIENT is fixed at 500mg, about half the total calcium supplied by the average diet. Children and women who are pregnant or breast-feeding, moreover, should have up to 1200mg per day. However, calcium obtained through wholemeal BREAD and some other foods is not absorbed (see below).

The richest sources are CHEESE, MILK and the small FISH, whitebait, sprats and smelts. About 100g (3½oz) of skimmed milk will supply the total daily recommended intake. Other good sources of calcium include watercress, parsley, shellfish, herring, pilchards, soya flour and fruit gums. Hard WATER contains the mineral. It is also found in dark green VEGETABLES such as spinach and beet tops, but in these vegetables oxalic acid reduces the ABSORPTION of calcium, just as phytic acid does in wholewheat bread. It is added to white and brown flour by law, but not to wholewheat.

For calcium absorption to take place efficiently, VITAMIN D must be present in the gut as well as in the body. It acts with two HORMONES, calcitonin and parathormone, to maintain the correct amounts of calcium in bones, nerves, muscles and in the blood and other tissues. The delicate machinery maintaining this balance is not yet fully understood.

In bone, calcium combines with PHOSPHORUS to form apatite. The full-grown adult skeleton contains about 1200g of calcium. During childhood, when the bones are still growing, apatite is laid down at the ends of long bones where it slowly replaces cartilage. Throughout life, however, calcium and phosphorus are being removed from bones and redeposited in a continuous process of rebuilding and remodelling. In times of mineral shortages such as can occur during pregnancy, bone may become a major reservoir from which calcium is obtained for use in other tissues. If removal of calcium goes too far as sometimes occurs during ageing, the bones become brittle and more subject to fracture.

During childhood, vitamin-D deficiency causes inadequate calcium deposition in bone, the condition observed as rickets. In adults, a similar condition is called osteomalacia. There is evidence that healthy bone-building during childhood protects the adult against osteomalacia in the event of a temporary vitamin-D deficiency such as can occur in the sunless northern winters.

About 10g of calcium exist free in the adult body. In this form, it is a charged atom called an ion, and it is in this form that the mineral is needed for the proper functioning of nerve and muscle cells. If the amount of tissue calcium falls, it is withdrawn from bone, but if bone reserves also become depleted, both muscle and nerve cells may malfunction causing muscular twitch and tetany. Tetany can also occur because of a disease of the parathyroid which causes the gland to produce too much parathormone. The disease is usually treatable with vitamin D, but if the tetany persists, surgical removal of part of the gland may be necessary.

The free calcium in blood is also an essential factor in blood clotting. Without it, bleeding will persist though the familiar disease, haemophilia, has another cause.

Diets consistently low in calcium produce an adaptive response in the body. It manages to do with less, at least for a period of time that varies with the individual. If there is plenty of vitamin D and if food calcium eventually becomes available, non-pregnant adults can usually get by with less than the recommended daily intake.

Excess calcium is a threat only in cases of vitamin-D deficiency or parathyroid disease. Normally, the urine carries off any excess, but a few people have too much calcium in their urine, a disease called hypercalcuria. These people can develop kidney stones. If the stones are small, they may be passed after much pain, but larger stones may have to be removed surgically. The usual treatment to prevent stones is a low-calcium diet; for example, the patient avoids cheese and milk and drinks at least four pints of water a day.

Too much vitamin D may also create a calcium excess which is absorbed into the blood. It is then deposited in the linings of blood vessels and can cause potentially fatal blockages. On the other hand, hardening of the arteries or atherosclerosis is not usually caused by too much calcium (see CHOLESTEROL) though its actual aetiology is still controversial.

CALORIE

A unit of ENERGY obtained from food. The calorie is a measure of heat energy. One calorie is the amount of heat needed to raise the temperature of 1g of WATER by 1 degree C.

The common unit of energy measurement in food is the Calorie, with a capital C, which is 1000 calories (small c) or 1 kilocalorie (kcal). The International System of Units of heat energy uses the Joule (J) instead of the Calorie as the unit of measurement for the energy content of food. The Joule equals roughly 250 calories or 0.25 Calories; 1 Calorie equals 4.1855 J. Although the Joule, which is defined as the energy produced by 1 watt of electricity in one second, is now widely used by nutritional scientists, in this *Dictionary* food energy will be measured by the more familiar Calorie.

CANCER
Runaway multiplication of cells in one or more parts of the body which increasingly invade and starve normal tissue. Some cancers of the digestive tract are thought to be associated with aspects of diet.

The DIGESTIVE PROCESS takes place along 32 feet of pockets, bags and tubes, any part of which may become a site for cancer growth. For reasons that are by no means clear, cancers in the different organs occur with varying frequencies in different parts of the world. Cancers of the digestive tract are most common in the UK and the US (cancer of the colon), Ireland (stomach), central and Latin America (stomach), Siberia (stomach), Japan (stomach), northern Europe and parts of China (oesophagus, the tube connecting the throat and the stomach). It is reasonable to suppose that dietary differences explain the epidemiology of these cancers, but the problem is to show why eating or failing to eat a certain food causes cancer.

Some authorities believe that inadequate dietary FIBRE explains the high incidence of cancer of the colon in the UK and the US. Two kinds of evidence support the connection, but both are theoretical rather than experimental. Cancer of the colon is very rare in regions such as central Africa where the diet contains much more fibre. On the other hand, although the northern European diet is very similar to that of the UK, oesophagial cancer is more common there. It would appear that fibre cannot be the only aetiological factor.

In the second kind of evidence, a connection is sought between the relatively slow passage of food through the intestines when the diet is low in fibre and the occurrence of colon cancer. There is clinical evidence that slow passage is a cause of a common western digestive disorder, DIVER-TICULITIS. If the waste also causes cancer of the colon, it must be because dietary waste contains a cancer-causing substance and that carcinogen requires protracted contact with the intestinal lining to produce the cancer. Yet no carcinogen has yet been identified in food waste that might operate in the manner described.

There are three general theories of carcinogenesis: environmental, viral and immunological. None excludes the possibility that the other two types of cause might also be at work. All three theories attempt to explain the changes in ordinary cell function that lead to cancer. Any one or all of them could of course apply to cancers of the digestive tract.

Cells multiply by division. A single fertilized ovum becomes two, four, eight and so on. At first, any one of these cells seems to be able to become any part of the body, but this capability soon disappears. Within the first week of embryonic life, cells have somehow organized themselves into regions and specialized in function. For example, the forerunner cells of the brain and spinal cord have formed a neural tube by the end of the first week.

The factors governing specialization are unknown, but the machinery at work can be described. It is the genetic material within each cell, the chromosomes, large molecules containing the genes along their length. Every cell in each body has the same set of genes, half from the mother and half from the father. Within the first few days after fertilization, however, some of the genes stop functioning, or it is also possible that some genes that had not begun to act now do so. This would be the process underlying specialization. Each gene directs the biosynthesis of a PROTEIN. Nerve cells contain one set of proteins whereas blood cells contain another set. Many of them are identical between the two sets, but others are unique to nerves and to blood cells, respectively. The result is that the two cell types differ in appearance, function, NUTRIENT needs, life-span and so on. The body is made up of thousands of cell types all containing the same set of genes, but normally, different genes are functioning in different cell types.

In healthy cells, specialization cannot be reversed. A colon lining cell remains a colon lining cell until it dies. When it divides, it produces two new colon lining cells, no more and no less. Cancer cells differ from normal cells in that they have lost their specialization. Instead of forming two new cells in the lining of the colon, a colon lining cell that has become a cancer cell neither looks nor acts like a colon lining cell. What is more, it may divide more rapidly than its normal neighbour, and it may divide into three or four daughter cells rather than just two.

Again, the machinery underlying this change of state has been pinpointed. A chemical change called a mutation takes place in one gene out of the thousands each cell possesses. That changed gene directs biosynthesis of a new protein which disorders the cell. In two forms of cancer, the exact mutation has been identified. Neither is a cancer of the digestive tract, but one is a bladder cancer.

The three theories about the cause of cancer are designed to explain what produces the mutation. Possible environmental carcinogens include asbestos, coal-tar constituents, radioactivity (see also POISON, FOOD) and food constituents such as NITROSAMINES. Only one of these, radioactivity, has been shown experimentally to produce mutations that could cause cancer. The others are associated statistically with one or more forms of the disease. Thus, many more of the people who develop lung cancer once smoked than did not smoke. Artificial SWEETENERS such as SACCHARIN are associated statistically with cancer in rats but not in humans. In the case of fibre, no constituent of food waste has yet been connected with cancer even statistically.

Viruses can produce mutations in the genes of human cells. Specific viruses are believed to cause a form of leukaemia and another form of human cancer, Burkitt's lymphoma, but others may also be implicated. There is no evidence, however, that viruses in food have anything to do with cancers of the digestive tract.

The immunological theory is not an explanation of how the cancerous mutation is caused. It proposes reasons why cancer cells escape normal constraints on growth. Cancer cells contain at least one gene that differs from genes in normal cells. For that reason, their biochemistry is aberrant. Their enclosing membranes should contain molecules not found in the membranes of their normal neighbours. In this sense, they are foreign cells. As such, they should be attacked and destroyed by the body's natural immune defences against invaders (see ALLERGY, FOOD). No one knows why they are not, but the immunological theory suggests ways in which cancer cells could fool the immune defences. It is possible, moreover, that an environmental factor or a virus has been immune suppressive. Thus, nitrosamines in food might interfere with the immunological capability of the body, but there is no evidence to support this hypothesis.

In short, although epidemiological evidence suggests that cancer of the colon could be associated with a lack of dietary fibre, no one can say how this deficiency produces cancer cells. Not even a theory based on epidemiology can be advanced to explain other cancers of the digestive tract.

CARBOHYDRATE
In food, principally CELLULOSE, STARCH or SUGAR. Cellulose along with gums and other indigestible plant carbohydrates make up FIBRE. Starch and sugar are used by the body to make ENERGY. With FAT and PROTEIN, carbohydrate is one of the three main constituents of food.

Sugar is almost unique among foods in that it consists of only one NUTRIENT, carbohydrate. All other carbohydrate-containing foods also contain other nutrients. BREAD and potatoes are good examples. Carbohydrates in sugar are called 'empty CALORIES'; they can be dropped from the diet without risk to the supply of other nutrients.

Starch consists of thousands of sugar molecules chemically linked together to form chains. By itself, starch also contains empty calories, but it is rarely eaten alone. In plants, starch forms as a means of storing sugar which has been synthesized out of carbon dioxide and WATER using the energy from sunlight. The sugar in starch is maltose, a disaccharide (di = two + saccharide = sugar) consisting of two molecules of glucose, a mono- (i.e. one) saccharide. Pure glucose is uncommon in unprocessed food, though small amounts may be obtained from MEAT.

The DIGESTIVE PROCESS breaks down all carbohydrates to glucose and other monosaccharides. Only these simple sugars are absorbed through the intestinal walls. Inside the body, ENZYMES convert other monosaccharides to glucose which may be stored in cells throughout the body as GLYCOGEN, also called animal starch. When we need energy, glycogen is broken down so that the glucose becomes available to cells. In other words, the carbohydrates built up in plants using solar energy are broken down by animals as a source of heat and chemical energy with the release of carbon dioxide and water.

All carbohydrates provide about 4.1 Calories per gram. Almost exactly the same energy is obtained from protein. Excess carbohydrate may also be converted into fat for storage. Fat and carbohydrate both consist of carbon, hydrogen and oxygen, and can be converted into one another with the expenditure of energy. Similarly, carbohydrate and protein can be converted into one another although protein contains at least one other element, nitrogen. This interchangeability of the principal nutrients explains why diets can stress cutting down on protein (for example, BEVERLY HILLS DIET), fats (SCARSDALE) or carbohydrate (F-PLAN). Conversely, if the intake of fats and/or proteins is reduced, the dieter can eat more carbohydrate and still lose weight. However, because sugar is pure carbohydrate and can be dropped without other losses resulting, cutting down on carbohydrates is probably the simplest way to lose weight. If the carbohydrate is cellulose, for example, it is not digested and can be eaten with no effect on either weight or nutrition.

VEGETABLES, dairy foods, and fresh meat are low in

carbohydrates. EGGS, FISH, CHEESE, butter and cream contain almost none. The table lists some of the common sources of carbohydrate and shows the other nutrients in these foods:

Food	Carbohydrate (g)	Fat	Protein	Vitamins	Minerals
White bread (4 slices)	49.7	+	++	++	++
Cream crackers (about 8)	68.3	++	++	+	++
Fruit cake (1 slice)	58.3	++	+	+	+
Spaghetti, boiled (4 tbsp)	26	+	+	+	+
Eating apple (1 large)	11.9	t	+	++	+
Banana (1 large)	19.2	+	+	++	++
Instant coffee (1 cup, black)	11	0	+	t	++
Mars bar	66.5	++	+	t	++

t = trace.
+ = small amounts.
++ = substantial part of daily requirement.

DIABETES is a disorder of carbohydrate uptake by cells. The METABOLISM of fat and protein is also disrupted. One important treatment for all diabetics is a LOW-CARBOHYDRATE DIET. EXERCISE is also widely recommended. Although carbohydrates are not directly associated with disease of the heart or circulation, foods containing them can cause OBESITY which puts a serious strain on the heart. Sugar may also play some role in hardening of the arteries (atherosclerosis). A low-carbohydrate diet may be healthful, moreover, because it helps to control excess CHOLESTEROL and LOW-DENSITY LIPOPROTEINS. In any case, as noted above, cutting carbohydrate intake is probably the simplest form of weight control for most healthy adults.

CELEVAC ®
A SLIMMING AID and a laxative.

Celevac is a bulk filler. It consists of an indigestible CARBOHYDRATE, methylcellulose, which swells when it is eaten. Thus, it adds bulk to the diet and is supposed to have the effect of filling the stomach. The evidence that it reduces appetite is controversial, but it can cause flatulence, abdominal distension and even intestinal obstruction.

Celevac is not addictive. However, it is sold only on prescription.

See also CELLUCON, NILSTIM.

CELLUCON ®
A SLIMMING AID and laxative. It contains the same chemical (methylcellulose) as CELEVAC and NILSTIM, with the same effects, but it is produced by a different company.

CELLULOSE
The main component of food FIBRE.

Cellulose forms the cell walls of plants but it is not found in animals. Cooking softens cellulose so that NUTRIENTS within the cells became accessible to the DIGESTIVE PROCESS. For this reason, raw VEGETABLES may actually provide less nutritional content than those that have been cooked, but raw vegetables add proportionately more to dietary fibre.

Cellulose is a CARBOHYDRATE consisting of a long chain of molecules of the SUGAR, glucose. ENZYMES to digest cellulose occur in the stomachs of horses, cows, sheep and other ruminants but not in humans.

In a slightly modified form, cellulose is a SLIMMING AID and laxative called a bulk filler (see CELEVAC, CELLUCON, NILSTIM). It is also a major constituent of important non-food products such as cloth, paper, plastics and explosives.

CEREAL
1. The seeds of grasses large enough to be milled and handled economically. 2. A processed food usually eaten for breakfast in western countries and derived from 1, plus other foods including SUGAR, dried FRUIT and other desiccated substances.

The grasses most commonly used as cereals are barley, maize (corn), millet, oats, rice, rye and wheat. TAPIOCA from the root of the cassava may be called a cereal and replaces cereals as the main element of diet in west Africa.

In the rest of the world outside the western nations, cereals properly defined are still the largest component of diet.

This entry will describe:

1. Barley	6. Rye
2. Maize	7. Wheat
3. Millet	8. Cereal nutrients
4. Oats	9. Dried breakfast cereal
5. Rice	

1. Barley (*Hordeum*), with rice and wheat, is the oldest known cereal. Carbonized remains have been found in Neolithic artifacts from Egypt and dated between 6000 and 5000 B.C. Barley was used by the Romans as a standard of weight, 24 seeds to the ounce. Similarly, in 1495, Henry VII made wheat grains into the standard of both weight and volume.

Three types of barley exist. In Britain and the US, the most common is the hulled two-row type. Six-row barley was common in early European history and is now found in India and the Middle East. Hull-less barley is grown in south-east Asia.

In the west, barley is used mainly as animal food. Some goes into the malting and brewing of BEER, manufacture of pearl barley, baby foods and COFFEE substitutes. For the NUTRIENTS in barley, see the table in section 8 of this entry, below.

2. Maize (*Zea mays*) originated in the Americas, the only cereal known to have done so. In the US, and increasingly in the UK, it is called corn. The maize seed, familiar from fresh corn on the cob and tinned corn, is the largest cereal seed.

Three types are grown. Field corn is used primarily as animal feed. Sweet corn has more sugars than the other types and is the common food corn. Flour types are softer. They are milled for cornflour or the coarser corn meal.

Like wheat, maize foods take many forms. In the UK and the US, cornflakes are popular. The tortillas of central and South America are small, flat maize cakes. Cornmeal porridge is called polenta in Italy and Romania, ogi in Nigeria, cornmeal cakes in Kenya and hominy grits in parts of the US. Maize oil is the principal constituent of most cooking oils.

3. Millet is used primarily as animal food and birdseed in Britain and the United States. Throughout central Africa, it is an important human food, either as flour or in beer. In Nigeria, a fermented millet also makes ogi, and in Ethiopia, a bread called ingera.

The most important of the millets is sorghum (*Sorghum vulgare*), also called durra, jowar, Guinea corn, kaffir corn, Indian millet and Egyptian corn. It is depicted in Egyptian tomb paintings from 2200 B.C. and today grows practically everywhere. The plant resists drought and tolerates very poor soil.

4. Oats (*Avena*) is also primarily an animal feed. However, in the UK and the US, it is popular as porridge. Oatcakes of oat and wheat flour, sugar and treacle are a Scottish speciality. Cicero recommended oats for medicinal purposes. Oat flour contains ANTIOXIDANTS which makes it a useful cereal mixer, and it is widely used in baby foods. Oats have a bitter taste which can be removed by heating.

Oats grow in cool, moist areas like northern Europe, parts of the US and Canada in poorer soil than is needed for wheat.

5. Rice (*Oriza sativa*) is eaten more widely by more people than any other cereal. It is the staple food of half the world's population. More than half the world's crop is consumed on the farms that grow it.

Rice was first mentioned in Chinese records of 2800 B.C., and China still grows the largest amount followed by India, Bangladesh, Japan and Thailand. Typically, rice is a swamp cereal grown in water in temperatures averaging about 22°C. Two crops a year are common. About 10 per cent of the world harvest consists of upland rice grown on hilly ground in parts of Africa and Asia. The most expensive cereal in the market is American wild rice, a different species also known as Indian or Tuscarora rice. It was traditionally farmed by American Indians. Its PROTEIN content is higher than that of most other cereals, and it contains more of the essential AMINO ACIDS.

Most rice is cooked by boiling or frying and forms the basis of numerous dishes: risotto, paella, pilau, curry, rice pudding and so on. In Japan, rice is fermented to make sake.

6. Rye (*Secale*) grows better in cooler climates than other cereals. It is used mainly as animal feed, but human consumption takes several forms. Rye BREAD is baked from a variable mixture of wheat and rye flour, and the product ranges from heavy, black Westphalian pumpernickel to light Swedish crispbread. Rye is fermented for whisky (US), gin (Holland) and beer (USSR). The use of rye for human consumption is declining, however, because it is hard to store rye grain which tends to sprout in the ear.

Ergot, the covering of a fungus, *Claviceps purpura*, can infect all cereals but is most common on rye. Its constituent drugs cause hallucinations, circulatory disorders and the loss of fingers and toes because of blood poisoning. Known in Europe as St Anthony's Fire, ergotism was as common as plague in the middle ages. In the UK, it last appeared in 1930, but in France, 300 inhabitants of one village were stricken as recently as 1951. Fifty became insane and three died.

7. Wheat may be one of several species. The most common and certainly the most important is bread wheat (*Triticum vulgare*). Different wheats are milled to produce flour of different 'strength', i.e. gluten content. Strong flour comes principally from Canadian spring wheat. It has a high protein content, 10 to 12 per cent, and therefore, a strong gluten content. Medium strength flour contains slightly less protein (9–11 per cent), and the gluten is softer. It comes from American winter wheat, Australian, Argentinian and strong European wheats. Most all-purpose flour for home baking is made from medium flour. Soft flour containing 7 to 9 per cent protein is best for baking cakes and biscuits but is less satisfactory for bread. English wheat is of the soft variety as is some other European and Australian wheat. Bread flour is usually a mixture of flour strengths called a mixed grist in which medium flour accounts for 30 to 40 per cent.

8. Cereal nutrients in some common products:

Nutrients per 100mg	Whole-meal wheat* flour	Pearl barley, boiled	Corn-flour	Oatmeal, raw	Rye flour	Polished rice, boiled
Calories	318	120	354	401	335	123
Protein (g)	13.2	2.7	0.6	12.4	8.2	2.2
Fat (g)	2	0.6	0.7	8.7	2	0.3
Carbohydrate (g)	65.8	27.6	92	72.8	75.9	29.6
Sodium (mg)	3	1	52	33	0	6
Potassium (mg)	360	40	61	370	410	38
Magnesium (mg)	140	7	7	110	92	4
Phosphorus (mg)	340	70	39	380	360	34
Calcium (mg)	35	3	15	55	32	1
Iron (mg)	4	0.2	1.4	4.1	2.7	0.2
Vitamins:						
B_1 (mg)	0.46	trace	trace	0.5	0.4	0.01
B_2 (mg)	0.08	trace	trace	0.1	0.22	0.01
B_3 (mg)	8.1	trace	trace	3.8	2.6	0.9
B_6 (mg)	0.5	trace	trace	0.12	0.35	trace
Folic acid (microg)	82	trace	trace	71	109	3
Vitamin E (mg)	1	trace	0	0.8	0.8	trace

* For milled flours, see BREAD.
Cereals contain no vitamin A, D, C or B_{12}.

The PHOSPHORUS in wheat and rice is present mainly as phytic acid which binds CALCIUM, IRON and MAGNESIUM, making the minerals unavailable as nutrients. Phytic acid is found mainly in the outer layers of the cereal grain, however, so that although white and brown bread and polished rice contain less calcium and iron than unmilled varieties, they also contain less phytic acid. Their calcium and iron are, therefore, more available for ABSORPTION.

9. Dried breakfast cereals are manufactured from wheat, maize, oats or rice by processes which reduce water and increase sugar content. For example, whereas 100g (3½oz) of wheat bran contain 8.3g of water and 3.8g of sugar, 'All Bran' has 2.3g of water and 15.4g of sugar. Incidentally, there is less dietary fibre in 'All Bran' than there is in wheat bran. 'Puffed Wheat' contains less sugar than other popular brands of dried cereal such as 'Cornflakes', 'Rice Crispies' and MUESLI. In part because of the dried fruit in the mixture, muesli has more added sugar than any other popular brand, and contrary to popular belief, it provides less dietary fibre (7.4g/100g) than some other cereals. Minerals and vitamins are added to all dried cereals but, except for 'Grapenuts', this does not include vitamins A, B_{12} and D. Vitamin C is also omitted, perhaps because breakfasts are supposed to begin with a fruit juice anyway. All popular breakfast cereals contain more CALORIES than the cereals from which they are manufactured.

CHEESE

A natural product of sour MILK produced from the milk solids curdled after removal of the watery whey. Cheese can be made from the milk of any animal. Its FLAVOUR and consistency depend upon which milk is used and on the manufacturing methods. In general, the longer the curds are allowed to sour, the harder the cheese.

Though it is a rich and widely available source of NUTRIENTS, milk has two serious drawbacks: without expensive and technically difficult storage or processing, it goes off quickly, and most adults lose some of their ability to digest milk because they no longer produce adequate amounts of lactase, an ENZYME that helps to break down the milk SUGAR, lactose. Cheese and YOGHURT are easier to digest because the lactose has been fermented, thus producing lactic acid which changes milk PROTEIN so that it hardens. This is the process known as curdling.

Legend has it that cheese was discovered by an Arab who was carrying goat's milk in a bag made from a sheep's stomach. The sun's heat turned the milk by encouraging bacteria to split the lactose for their food, and an enzyme, rennin, in the sheep's stomach caused the curdling. Rennin, incidentally, is a general term for this enzyme: when it comes from the fourth stomach of a calf, it is called rennet. (Yet another enzyme, renin, affects blood pressure but has nothing to do with digestion.) Whether or not the legend is true, however, it illustrates an important advance in food technology that was made by many tribes in many different places.

Cheese manufacture begins with the addition to milk of rennin, additional bacteria or a little lactic acid to form curd. The curds are heated and cut to release whey and then seeded with bacteria or a fungus selected on the basis of the product required. For example, the fungus, Penicillium (not the *Penicillium notatum* which produces penicillin but a relative), plays a role in the manufacture of Stilton and other blue cheeses. The mass is placed in a mould and fermented under carefully controlled temperature and humidity.

Cottage and cream cheeses may be used almost as soon as the curd is formed. Processed cheeses are made by combining several different cheeses in amounts selected to determine taste, consistency and melting time. Food ADDITIVES are used in unprocessed as well as processed cheeses. They include EMULSIFIERS, PRESERVATIVES and spices. LECITHIN is the main emulsifier though others may be employed in cheese manufacture. The main preservatives are NISIN, found naturally in some cheeses, and sorbic acid.

Like milk, cheese is an excellent source of ENERGY. For example, Cheddar contains three times the CALORIES found in the same weight of BREAD. Its Calories come primarily from FAT. Cheese contains very little CARBOHYDRATE and varying amounts of PROTEIN. Hard cheeses are richest in protein which amounts to about 25 per cent by weight of Cheddar. Cheddar and Parmesan are excellent sources of CALCIUM, but soft cheeses contain less. With the exception of cottage and cream cheese, SALT content is fairly high. If cottage and curd cheese are made with skimmed milk, they have less fat and fewer Calories than other cheeses, but cream cheese and cheeses made with added cream, like Stilton, are much higher in Calorie content.

The following table summarizes some nutrients in 100g (3½oz) of some popular cheeses:

	Camembert	Cheddar	Edam	Stilton	Cottage	Cream	Processed	Spread
Calories	300	406	304	462	96	439	311	283
Protein (g)	22.8	26	24.4	25.6	13.6	3.1	21.5	18.3
Fat (g)	23.2	33.5	22.9	40	4	47.4	25	22.9
Carbohydrate (g)	trace	trace	trace	trace	1.4	trace	trace	0.9
Minerals:								
Sodium (mg)	1410	610	980	1150	450	300	1360	1170
Potassium (mg)	110	120	160	160	54	160	82	150
Calcium (mg)	380	800	740	360	60	98	700	510
	17	25	28	27	6	10	24	25
Vitamins:								
A (microg)	215	310	215	370	32	385	240	180
B_1 (mg)	0.05*	0.04	0.04	0.07	0.02	0.02	0.02	0.02
B_2 (mg)	0.6	0.5	0.4	0.3	0.19	0.14	0.29	0.24
B_3† (mg)	6	6	6	6	4	1.5	5	4
B_6 (mg)	0.2	0.08	0.08	0	0.01	0.01	0	0
B_{12} (microg)	1.2	1.5	1.4	0	0.5	0.3	0	0
Folic acid (microg)	60	20	20	0	9	5	2	0
D (microg)	0.18	0.26	0.18	0.31	0.02	0.28	0.15	0.13
E (mg)	0.6	0.8	0.8	1	0	1	0	0

* Rind of Camembert only: 0.5 mg.
† Approximate values.

Cheese is easily digested. The feeling of fullness that a cheese meal imparts – presumably the foundation for the popular impression that it is hard to digest and causes dreams – may derive from the fact that high fat content tends to delay passage from the stomach to the small intestine.

Its uses are, of course, immensely varied, and it is safe to say that in too many households, cheese dishes are undervalued. To keep cheese from hardening when it is heated, it may be grated and mixed with a little milk, cornflour or mustard. In some processed cheeses this mixture has already been made.

Camembert, Cheddar, Stilton and some less popular cheeses contain significant amounts of an AMINO ACID, tyramine, which cannot be used by the body until it has been converted to tyrosine. The conversion requires a group of enzymes called monoamine oxidases. Certain antidepressant drugs inhibit these enzymes. If the patient then eats a cheese rich in tyramine, the amino acid builds up in the system causing headache and a rise in blood pressure which can be serious. Tyramine is also a constituent of beans, BEER and WINE, some MEAT and YEAST extracts and YOGHURT. Your doctor will normally warn you about these foods if you are using antidepressants.

CHELATING AGENT See SEQUESTRANT

CHLORINE
One of the two constituents of table SALT, the other being SODIUM. A small amount of chlorine is taken in from chlorinated WATER. In BREAD manufacture, chlorine dioxide is a permitted ADDITIVE and acts as an improver.

Salt is so pervasive in living things that a chlorine deficiency is unheard of apart from sodium deficiencies. Like salt, excess chlorine is secreted in sweat and urine.

The adult body contains about 70g of chlorine, most of it dissolved in the fluid surrounding cells. It is essential for the proper functioning of nerve and muscle cells and is used by cells in the stomach which synthesize hydrochloric acid. In the body, chlorine takes the form of chloride, a negative ion in solution.

Chlorine is a halogen, one of four gases that form sodium salts. The others are IODINE, FLUORINE and bromine.

CHOLESTEROL
A controversial constituent of many foods. Some authorities, particularly doctors in the US, maintain that excess cholesterol causes hardening of the arteries and heart disease, but the British medical profession tends to reject any

simple connection between cholesterol consumption and heart disease (see also LIPID, LOW-DENSITY LIPOPROTEIN).

The most common food sources are EGG yolk, butter, CHEESE and liver. By avoiding these foods, one's daily intake of cholesterol can be much reduced. In fact, we need none at all from food. Our bodies manufacture cholesterol. Synthesis takes place in the liver. Cholesterol is a fat-like molecule used by the body to build certain HORMONES including the sex hormones, BILE and the white sheaths that surround and protect many nerve cells. Cholesterol is far too important for the body to leave its supply to food availability or the whims of fashion.

On average, our bodies contain 140g of cholesterol of which 4 to 6g are found circulating in the blood. In some people, especially those who are older, the amount of cholesterol in the blood tends to rise. It may then contribute to the roughening and hardening of blood vessels, but the relationship between circulatory disease and dietary intake is disputed for two reasons. First, the body determines how much cholesterol it needs at any time in accordance with its metabolic (see METABOLISM) state. Second, evidence now points to another possible culprit, also a fat-like molecule called low-density lipoprotein. In any case, it appears to be the amount of these fatty substances in the blood, not the amount absorbed from food, that affects the circulation.

Nevertheless, low-fat, high-fibre and VEGETARIAN diets are associated with a reduction in the death rate from heart disease, particularly in the US and Scandinavia. The dietary changes may themselves be a reflection of tension-reducing changes in life-style which improve the general health of those who undertake them, however. For example, business executives who realize that their life-style may produce high health hazards may not only alter their diet but also increase their EXERCISE and sleep.

COELIAC DISEASE
1. A hereditary disorder of the DIGESTIVE PROCESS principally seen in early childhood. 2. A very similar disease

with no known genetic factor is now diagnosed in a growing number of adults aged over sixty in England, Wales and parts of the US.

In the usual childhood form of coeliac disease, the patient fails to absorb FATS including the fat-soluble VITAMINS, A, D, E and K, and some MINERALS. The children develop anaemia, probably because of an IRON shortage, and rickets because of vitamin D MALABSORPTION.

The cause of the disease is unknown. The patient is sensitive to GLUTEN, a PROTEIN found in wheat and rye flour and to a lesser extent in barley and oats (see CEREAL). Often the first symptoms are irritability and poor growth. A cure will usually follow rigid exclusion of gluten from the diet, but if the symptoms have been present too long, the intestinal villi, the organs through which ABSORPTION takes place, may be damaged. The child will probably be hospitalized until the intestinal lining has regenerated. In unusual cases, however, coeliac disease can be fatal.

Maize, rice and potatoes are gluten-free. The patient will also thrive on fresh MEAT, FISH, dairy products, VEGETABLES and FRUIT. On the other hand, many CONVENIENCE FOODS contain gluten. Parents may obtain dietary advice for their children from: The Coeliac Society, P.O. Box 181, London NW2 2QY.

In Britain, coeliac disease affects about one child in 2000. The child may grow out of the gluten intolerance, but symptoms of the disease can persist insidiously in what doctors call sub-clinical form. In such cases, the child may become anaemic. Adults with sub-clinical coeliac disease suffer from osteomalacia, a vitamin-D deficiency disease akin to rickets. Adults who develop the disease will probably have to follow a gluten-free diet permanently.

COFFEE
A beverage drunk hot or cold and with or without MILK, cream, SUGAR and various alcoholic drinks. Strong black coffee made with a tablespoon of ground coffee beans in a half-pint of nearly-boiling WATER contains a little POTASSIUM, traces of VITAMIN B_3, about 150mg of CAFFEINE and less than two CALORIES.

Because of the caffeine, coffee is a stimulant. For most of us, four cups a day, black or white, is probably enough if we are to avoid 'coffee nerves'. People with heart disorders or other chronic conditions should consult their doctors about safe limits. Coffee and TEA tend to be more stimulating for children, and the younger they are, the less they should drink.

The botanical name *Coffea arabica* was given to the plant because coffee came to Europe in the sixteenth century from Arabia via Egypt. It appears to be native to Ethiopia and Angola. Coffee growing was introduced into India and central east Africa by the British and into Latin America by the Spanish and Portuguese.

At the beginning of PROCESSING, the coffee beans are dried and the hulls removed mechanically. They are then roasted and packed either before or after grinding. Instant coffee is prepared by spray- or freeze-drying the prepared coffee infusion. It contains less potassium, vitamin B_3 and caffeine than fresh coffee. However, the decaffeinated drink is made from fresh beans which have been soaked in organic solvents or weak ACIDS or alkalis (see BASE). The treated beans are dried and roasted in the same way as fresh beans. By law, decaffeinated coffee must contain less than 0.1 per cent caffeine or about 2mg per cup.

Coffee substitutes such as chicory and figs contain no caffeine. French coffee made with chicory must contain 51 per cent coffee by weight. Viennese coffee made with figs is 85 per cent coffee. Coffee essences are concentrated infusions plus SUGAR, PRESERVATIVES and EMULSIFIERS.

COLOUR, FOOD
A quality of all natural foods derived from pigments such as chlorophyll (green), carotene (orange, as in carrots) or beetroot red. Pigments in our bodies include the haemoglobin in red blood cells. (Haemoglobin, of course, gives colour to MEAT.)

Processed foods often have colour added to make them more appealing to the eye. For example, peas tend to lose their colour when they are canned, so colour is added;

different batches of jam vary in colour, so artificial colouring is used to achieve uniformity. Different cultures expect foods to have different colours, moreover. Some Chinese sauces contain a bright red which makes them more attractive to the Chinese who created them but looks artificial and unappetizing to the western eye.

The coal-tar dyes are the most popular with food manufacturers because very small amounts produce lasting effects. However, the coal-tar dyes are suspected causes of CANCER. They are chemically related to elements in tobacco smoke, and evidence from experiments on animals shows that the dyes can cause cancer under certain conditions. Attempts are being made by manufacturers, therefore, to replace them with colours of different origin. Most of these are also synthetic of course.

Food colours are the most controversial of all ADDITIVES not only because many contain potential health hazards but also because they are unnecessary and raise marketing problems of their own. Certainly, added colours give no nutritional benefits to the food. What is more, different people respond differently to colours. It has been shown that one colour is unlikely to satisfy all markets, although manufacturers may try to meet this problem by using different colours for the same product. Yet these objections to the contrary notwithstanding, many foods of real importance might sell less well without added colour. For example, the market for brown BREAD might be significantly smaller if caramel, a natural colourant and the usual additive, was not used.

In the UK, the Food Additives and Contaminants Committee reported on colour additives in 1979. It recommended acceptance of about forty substances either with or without qualifications, or provisionally for a period of five years during which safety tests were to be continued. Only four dyes fell into the fully approved group whereas sixteen of the twenty-one non-dyestuffs have been recommended without qualification. Current UK regulations forbid the addition of colour to raw or unprocessed meat, game, POULTRY, FISH, FRUIT, VEGETABLES, TEA, COFFEE, coffee products, condensed or dried MILK. The 1979 report also recommended that current UK practice withholding colour additives from foods manufactured for infants and young children should become an official regulation. The report recommended that the manufacture of caramel or burnt SUGAR, the most common colouring agent, should be standardized. (Caramel is the only colouring permitted in bread.) A different agent, Brown FK (E151; see Appendix II), is used to colour kippers.

It is worth noting that unlike added colours, natural food colours change during cooking. For example, muscle PROTEIN in meat changes from red to brown and chlorophyll, from bright to dark green. Bicarbonate of soda or other mild alkalis will preserve the green, but they destroy VITAMIN C. Heat turns sugar brown. Substances called flavones in white vegetables (e.g. cauliflower) yellow during boiling unless an acid-containing substance such as VINEGAR is added to the WATER. Anthocyanins that give the red colour to cabbage turn blue in alkaline cooking water, but this process can be reduced somewhat by adding a little vinegar. The flavones in some fruits and vegetables brown in the air, a change that is due to the release of ENZYMES when the food is peeled or cut. Thus, if the food you are preparing for dinner does not change colour in the process, it probably contains synthetic additives.

COMFREY

(*Symphitum officianalis*) A common weed in early summer growing to a height of three feet with large, hairy green leaves and spikelets of white flowers. Eaten cooked or in salad, it supplies VITAMIN B_{12}, a rare constituent of VEGETABLES. However, its use in salads must be watched because a touch from hairs on older and larger leaves causes inflammation and itching of the skin and mucous membranes in the mouth.

Also called knit-bone because it is reputed to assist in that process, the sap of comfrey has been used in ointments to treat aches and sprains and in elixirs for diverse complaints. The plant contains allantoin, an alkaloid which encourages proliferation of cells in both skin and bone. This drug may well provide a foundation for its ancient reputation. Allantoin is also secreted by maggots and may explain their former use to keep wounds clean. However, no scientifically-controlled tests of comfrey (or maggots) have established its real value for any of these applications.

COMPLAN ®

A SLIMMING AID, but a food and not a drug. The package calls Complan a 'complete meal you drink' (see also SLENDER). Used alone, Complan provides a VERY LOW CALORIE DIET, containing 444 Calories per 100g (3½oz). The recommended meal consists of three or four dessert spoons or about 100g dissolved in a mug of water.

Complan contains dried skimmed MILK, vegetable FAT and various other components. It supplies adequate CARBOHYDRATE, fat and PROTEIN, a range of MINERALS including CALCIUM, copper, IRON, manganese, PHOSPHORUS, POTASSIUM, SODIUM and zinc and all VITAMINS.

CONVENIENCE FOOD

Manufactured or processed food which can be prepared rapidly and easily served. Perhaps the oldest are dried breakfast CEREALS and tinned soups, but the term covers FISH fingers, packaged MEAT pies and pre-cooked, presliced meat, instant puddings, cake mixes, TV dinners and RICE or noodle dishes packaged in a metal or plastic bowl to which the consumer merely adds hot WATER. By far the most elaborate convenience foods are the standard meals served by every airline.

The word 'convenience' has long been used in advertising by food processors, but the phrase itself is first listed in the *Oxford English Dictionary* from an article in *The Economist* dated 2 December 1961. Of course there is no more 'convenient' food than the MILK of a nursing mother. Still, convenience foods have acquired an image of nutritional inferiority which is often justified.

The loss of NUTRIENTS during PROCESSING is no greater than in home cooking, but the necessary reheating further reduces VITAMIN content. Also the ingredients of these packaged foods are often stored for longer periods than in the home, causing greater nutrient loss. ADDITIVES restore some of these losses, but one Australian study showed that on average a range of processed convenience foods contained 55 per cent less PROTEIN and 60 per cent less vitamin B$_1$ than similar foods prepared in a domestic kitchen.

CUCUMBER
(*Cucumus sativus*) This green, gourd-like VEGETABLE requires moisture but will grow in remarkably infertile soil. For centuries, it has been regarded as a cleanser for the skin and internal organs, perhaps because it is cool and pleasant to touch. Apart from their obvious value in salads, cucumbers form a suitable part of every diet whether the dietary regimen stresses CARBOHYDRATES, FATS or PROTEINS. Cucumbers are commonly cooked and served as vegetables in the Soviet Union and China.

One hundred grams (3½oz) of cucumber, a hefty portion, contain a mere 10 CALORIES. They have very little carbohydrate (1.8g per 100g) and only a trace of fat, but adequate amounts of CALCIUM, PHOSPHORUS and POTASSIUM plus small quantities of other MINERALS. Their protein, VITAMIN and FIBRE content are also low. No one can survive on a diet of cucumbers. Because it virtually lacks energy and protein, anyone eating cucumber as part of a shock diet should also eat FRUIT which helps to combat the bloating and constipation that are liable to be caused by the lack of fibre in cucumbers.

See also BEVERLY HILLS DIET, F-PLAN DIET.

D

DANDELION
(*Taraxacum officianalis*) The familiar, jagged-leaved weed with its bright yellow flowers and balls of grey seeds was once called piss-a-bed. Only the bitterness of the leaves

stands in the way of more widespread use of this valuable VEGETABLE. Its NUTRIENT content is roughly the same as spinach.

Small amounts in salad add a piquancy which many people enjoy. The flowers can be fermented, with a loss of most of the nutrients, of course, for a slightly bitter WINE. They may also be mixed with other flowers and FRUIT before FERMENTATION to vary the FLAVOUR of the wine. Dandelion roots are dried and stored for grinding and brewing into dandelion COFFEE. Indeed, it is possible to buy ready-ground dandelion coffee powder.

The reputed curative powers of dandelion are less certain than its nutritional value, but for centuries it has been used as an antacid and to treat anaemia, high blood pressure and other more serious conditions. Dandelion is also said to increase longevity.

DIABETES

A potentially fatal disease affecting the body's use of CARBOHYDRATES, FATS and PROTEINS and characterized by the appearance of too much SUGAR in the blood and urine. Though there is a familial tendency to diabetes, its cause is unknown. All diabetics require a rigorous carbohydrate-controlled diet and regular EXERCISE.

In addition to excess sugar, symptoms and signs of diabetes may include weight loss, apathy, thirst, itching, changes in eye function, loss of feeling in the extremities, boils, heart disorders, and in cases where blood sugar has risen too high or fallen too low following an insulin injection, coma and death. All of these symptoms and effects reflect either an inadequate supply of insulin or a failure to use the HORMONE normally. Insulin causes cells to take up sugar in the form of glucose from the blood. Either the glucose is used immediately to produce ENERGY, or it is stored in the form of GLYCOGEN. Insulin may also influence the body's ability to form protein from AMINO ACIDS. In this way, the hormone is required for both growth and maintenance.

In the absence of insulin, cells starve in the midst of

plenty: despite the presence of glucose in the blood and body fluids, cells seem incapable of absorbing it. In order to maintain their functions, the glucose-starved cells convert fat and protein to energy-producing carbohydrate. This desperate makeshift itself uses up energy and eats up the body. Fat breakdown, moreover, produces substances called KETONES in amounts that disturb the ACID-BASE balance of body fluids, further compromising normal METABOLISM.

The patient must reduce carbohydrate intake and exercise regularly as a means of controlling excess sugar. There are two distinctive types of diabetes, however: early- and late-onset. In the former, insulin is seldom being produced by the patient's pancreas, or if it is, the amounts are inadequate. Insulin will be injected. In late-onset diabetes, the patient is often producing adequate amounts of insulin which are failing to function for some reason. All diabetic diets aim to keep blood glucose in balance with the available insulin, whether natural or injected. Insulin cannot be given orally because it is a protein and would be quickly destroyed by the DIGESTIVE PROCESS. When the patient has some insulin of his or her own, diet and exercise alone may control the disease. When insulin is required, the problem is to balance dietary carbohydrate and the injected hormone. Unusual exercise, stress and illness can disrupt a carefully-developed regimen. Each diabetic patient is walking a tight-rope of his or her own design. Diet and insulin dose, if one is needed, must be determined by a doctor, perhaps with the help of a professional dietitian, using trial and error. The object is to supply enough sugar to supply energy and no more.

To make control easier through diet, allowable carbohydrate is usually divided into three or four meals a day. Once the proper balance has been discovered, the patient may trade off carbohydrate-containing dishes but only on a carefully measured basis. For example, if the patient is allowed 100g (3½oz) of carbohydrate per day and this is customarily divided into 10g portions, then he or she may obtain 10g from a tablespoon (35g) of boiled RICE, half a large banana (weighing 50g), 50g (2oz) of baked beans or two level teaspoons of white or brown sugar. Protein intake may not require regulation. The patient's need for MINERALS and VITAMINS will be the same as that of a healthy person of similar age, occupation and weight. However, fats will also be restricted because of the possible connection between CHOLESTEROL and LOW-DENSITY LIPO-PROTEIN in the blood and circulatory diseases.

Early-onset diabetes occurs before the age of twenty and is usually the more serious illness. In most cases, patients need insulin injections for the rest of their lives. Late-onset diabetes seldom occurs before the age of thirty and usually after forty. The patient is often overweight. His or her pancreas may produce even more insulin than normal, and in any case, insulin injections are useless in most cases. Synthetic drugs such as chlorpropamide (Diabinase) may help cells to utilize at least some of the naturally available insulin. Even in late-onset diabetes, however, a sudden failure of the insulin-producing cells in the islets of Langerhans within the pancreas can occur unpredictably. The patient will die without immediate, massive injections of insulin, and then the balancing process must be introduced just as in early-onset patients.

The full name of this baffling disease is diabetes mellitus (Greek: a passer through or syphon + sweet, honeyed). Another disease, diabetes insipidus, is characterized by excessive urination, dehydration and disruption of the ACID-BASE balance in body fluids. Neither insulin nor diet have an effect on diabetes insipidus though it can be treated with drugs.

DIET, BALANCED

Diet is the food we eat and not merely a programme designed for weight reduction. The idea of balance in diet developed early in this century as it became apparent that food contains a remarkable variety of NUTRIENTS serving many different purposes in the body's economy. A balanced diet is based on scientific data about body needs and recommends the minimum intake of MINERALS, PROTEIN and VITAMINS required to prevent deficiency diseases such as iron-deficiency anaemia, KWASHIORKOR (protein deficiency) or scurvy (vitamin-C deficiency). A balanced diet will also include CARBOHYDRATE and FAT to provide the ENERGY for living, working and reproduction, but because the only deficiency disease associated with inadequate intake of energy-producing foods is starvation, it has been taken for granted that people who have enough to eat, eat enough carbohydrate and fat.

Doctors and nutritionists have known for years that in the affluent nations of Europe and north America, the old notion of a balanced diet based on minimum daily requirements is no longer relevant to real health hazards: degenerative diseases related to diet such as bad teeth, DIABETES, OBESITY and cardiovascular diseases. Very few people in Britain suffer from scurvy, and no one dies from it. On the other hand, the death rate from heart disease in Scotland and Northern Ireland is the highest in the world, and the poorer you are, the greater your risk. The total bill for all diet-related diseases in the United Kingdom in 1980 was conservatively estimated at £660 million. Heart disease and dental caries are not deficiency diseases. Indeed, they are more closely related to eating too much, or at least too much of the very food constituents that are ignored by recommended mimimums: fats and carbohydrates, in particular, SUGAR.

The old ideas of a balanced diet are still scientifically correct. You must have adequate protein, vitamins and minerals in your diet. But the old ideas fail to take into consideration the changes in income and in what we eat which have taken place during the last century. Only 15 per cent of what we spend on food today pays for raw products as opposed to processed and manufactured foods. Until well into the present century, our fat consumption represented less than 30 per cent of our diets whereas now it is over 40 per cent. New foods – hamburgers, pastas and indeed YOGHURT, among others – have become a standard part of the British diet. Commercial hamburgers are made with fatty mince, and the white buns in which they are served contain little FIBRE. Though pasta has much to recommend it, it too has little fibre and in the sauces, usually too much fat. Yoghurt can be a safe and nutritious food if it is made with skimmed MILK and unsweetened, but most of the yoghurt sold contains added sugar and is made with whole milk. In the face of our changing eating habits, the idea of a balanced diet should now include safe maximums as well as required minimums.

The establishment of safe dietary guidelines recommending maximums is certainly desirable but, scientifically, it is not simple. We all differ in the work we do, our genetic makeup, our highly individual bundles of tastes. Yet these are the factors that determine what we eat. No disease, furthermore, can be blamed entirely on diet. Even tooth decay: some lucky children can eat sweets almost without limit and still have very few cavities. They are a tiny minority, but they demonstrate that other factors, both genetic and environmental, play a role in tooth decay. Nevertheless, statistical and hard experimental evidence link sugar consumption with dental caries. Similarly, both statistical and experimental evidence link fat consumption to cardiovascular disease, at least indirectly, and low-fibre diets are associated with bowel disorders. Changes in lifestyle affecting diet and EXERCISE among other factors have reduced heart disease-related deaths by 25 per cent in the United States and Australia since 1968. The need for new dietary guidelines can no longer be brushed aside.

In 1983, proposals for nutritional guidelines for the British were published by the National Advisory Committee on Nutrition Education (NACNE), the first comprehensive new proposals to be put forward since World War II. They fall under six broad headings: fats, sugar, SALT, energy, fibre and protein.

1. **Fats.** Reduction of total fat intake by 10 per cent from roughly 38 per cent of total CALORIES to 34 per cent. Saturated animal fats (see LIPID) which are believed to be more harmful, to be reduced by 15 per cent and polyunsaturated vegetable OILS to rise by roughly 25 per

cent. This rise is offset because our present diets include far more saturated animal fats, about 59g per day, than vegetable fats, about 14.5g per day.

The proposal means that in practice we should eat less high-fat foods. For adults, whole milk should be replaced by skimmed milk. Butter should be replaced with vegetable-based, butterfree MARGARINES. Cream and CHEESE make up a small proportion of most diets and should simply be watched. Perhaps most important, fat MEATS should be replaced by lean. Liver and offal as well as FISH and poultry are healthier sources of protein than sausages and hamburgers. Finally, use vegetable oils for cooking instead of butter.

2. Sugar. Sweet, white and deadly, it has been called. The NACNE proposals call for a 50 per cent reduction in average intake from 38kg (84lb) to 20kg (44lb) per year immediately and eventually to no more than 15kg per year. Such a reduction will require that food and SOFT DRINKS manufacturers either make their products less sweet or replace sugar with artificial SWEETENERS. Each of us can also reduce the amount of sugar we put into tea or coffee and on our breakfast CEREAL. FRUIT can sometimes replace pastries for desserts and between-meal snacks. In particular, the current trend towards the reduction of sugar given to children will often diminish their craving for sweets in adult life.

3. Salt. Ordinary table salt provides essential SODIUM and CHLORINE, but our needs are easily met. Excess salt causes the body to retain WATER contributing to overweight and blood circulation problems and placing an additional strain on the kidneys. Because we tend to consume far more salt than we need, it is recommended that our salt consumption be cut by 10 per cent. In practice, this means cutting down the salt you use in cooking or at the table by about one gram a day, a tiny amount. Again, it will be necessary for official bodies to ask food processors to play their role because they now contribute the largest part of the salt we eat.

4. Energy. Instead of cutting Calories, the NACNE proposals recommend that they remain the same, and that we increase our daily exercise. Because of the recommended fat and sugar reductions we are expected to enforce, however, we can eat more BREAD and potatoes, fruit and vegetables without increasing our Calorie intake. In fact, by cutting down on fats and sugar as specified above, our consumption of bread, potatoes, fruit and vegetables can rise by almost a third.

5. Fibre. If the additional bread is wholemeal, the increased bread consumption should contribute the equivalent of the recommended 25 per cent increase in dietary fibre, from about 20g at present to 25g a day.

6. Protein. No change in total protein consumption is recommended, but if we accept the other recommendations, our sources of protein will shift. We will be eating more fish and less fat meat, more bread, potatoes and other vegetables and less cheese.

The NACNE proposals also recommend a 10 per cent cut in our ALCOHOL consumption. Alcohol provides Calories with no other NUTRIENTS. For a person who drinks an average of two pints a day, the recommended reduction amounts to about a fifth of a pint or roughly two to three tablespoons a day, about 1½ pints per week.

If we accept these proposals and act on them, there should be immediate benefits for each of us as well as the long-range assurance that our children will be healthier than many of us have been. For example, an increase in fibre will help most people avoid constipation and may lower the risk from bowel CANCER and DIVERTICULITIS. But there are no miracle diets, the claims of some of the authors whose books are described in this *Dictionary* to the contrary notwithstanding. Diet is not by itself the cause of bowel cancer or heart disease. The NACNE proposals are designed to provide a better foundation for the national health. Of course, the familiar recommendations that we eat specified amounts of essential AMINO ACIDS, minerals and vitamins continue to be valid, too.

DIGESTIVE PROCESS

1. The breakdown of food into its constituent NUTRIENTS and waste by mechanical and chemical activity in the digestive tract. 2. The process described in 1, and the subsequent ABSORPTION of the nutrients into the body.

The digestive tract begins at the mouth and ends at the anus. Food in the mouth is mixed with saliva to form a ball or bolus. Swallowing sends this bolus into the back of the throat whence it enters the oesophagus, a long tube leading to the stomach. A process of wave-like motion called peristalsis in the walls of the oesophagus and the intestines propels the food through the entire 32 feet of the pouches and tubes that follow. After two to four hours of squeezing and mixing with gastric juice in the stomach, the food passes through the pyloric sphincter into the duodenum, the portion of the small intestine nearest the stomach. In the small intestine, itself about 27 feet long, the walls are lined with villi through which absorption takes place. Eight to nine hours after a meal, the remaining fluid, FIBRE, residues of BILE and digestive juices, mucus, dead cells from the lining of the digestive tract, bacteria and undigested nutrients enter the large intestine. There, further absorption of nutrients and WATER leaves the faeces.

Nutrients are, of course, those chemical constituents of food which can be utilized or stored for later use by body cells. The breakdown of food into nutrients begins in the mouth. Chewing begins the mechanical breakdown. Saliva not only lubricates the mouth and throat and encourages formation of the bolus, but it also contains the ENZYME, ptyalin or salivary amylase. Ptyalin begins the chemical breakdown of cooked starch to a SUGAR, maltose. This process can actually be tasted. If you chew bread for a minute or so, it should become sweet.

No digestion occurs in the oesophagus, but in the stomach, mechanical action of the stomach walls mixes the food with gastric juice. The two major constituents of gastric juice are the enzyme, pepsin, and hydrochloric acid. Both are synthesized on demand by cells in the stomach wall. Pepsin splits PROTEIN into smaller molecules. Hydrochloric acid continues the breakdown of food, especially by softening CELLULOSE and other indigestible constituents so that nutrients can be released and absorbed.

The release of gastric juice is governed in three ways: first, by the presence of food in the stomach. Second, food in the stomach plus the sight, taste and smell of food cause the brain to signal the stomach via the vagus nerve. Third, food in the stomach and duodenum stimulate other stomach-wall cells to synthesize a HORMONE, gastrin, which enters the blood and extends the time-span of the commands initiated by the first two regulators. Another hormone, enterogastrone, which is also produced by stomach wall cells in the presence of fat causes a decrease in the movements of the stomach wall and thus delays emptying. At least one more constituent of gastric juice plays a vital role in the digestive process: intrinsic factor is a protein without which VITAMIN B_{12} cannot be absorbed.

If you eat continuously, your stomach continues to work. There is nothing harmful in this because the stomach wall cells producing gastric juice can normally function indefinitely. Indeed, people who have ULCERS and some other diseases and those with stomachs made smaller by surgery usually do eat smaller amounts more frequently. However, the presence of food in the stomach does divert blood and some nutrients required elsewhere for ENERGY, and EXERCISE must be suitably regulated.

When they leave the stomach, small portions of food called chyme (pronounced with a hard 'ch') pass into the duodenum. There pancreatic juice and bile attack the chyme. Pancreatic juice consists of five enzymes synthesized in the pancreas and delivered by ducts to the intestines. Trypsin and chymotrypsinogen complete the breakdown of proteins into their constituent AMINO ACIDS. Pancreatic amylase (the same enzyme as ptyalin) and maltase complete the breakdown of carbohydrates to simple sugars. Lactase, present in the pancreatic juice of children, may be much reduced or completely missing in adults. It acts on the milk sugar, lactose. Lipase breaks down fats into their constituents (see LIPID). Note that the pancreas also contains groups of cells which synthesize hormones such as insulin (see DIABETES).

MINERALS, most vitamins and ALCOHOL are absorbed through the intestinal villi without further digestion. In the presence of phytic or oxalic acid (see BREAD, CALCIUM, VEGETABLE), mineral absorption may be reduced because these substances tend to bind the minerals chemically so that they cannot be absorbed. Vitamins A, D, E and K are soluble in fats and can only be absorbed in the presence of bile. Apart from these specific nutrients, all food is broken down to the sugars, glucose, galactose and fructose, amino acids and the constituents of fat before absorption.

The millions of bacteria that normally inhabit the digestive tract are either benign or positively beneficial. Those that contribute to our well-being supply B vitamins, amino acids and minerals to supplement what we obtain from food, and they utilize our waste for their own nutrition. Large or continuous doses of certain antibiotics and laxatives can kill significant numbers of the bacteria in the gut disrupting the digestive process and encouraging growth of bacteria which may be harmful.

Between 60 and 90 per cent of the faeces is water. Of the dry matter, about half is bacteria and the remainder consists of dead cells, unused digestive juice and undigested fibre and food waste. Faeces continue to be produced even during starvation.

Vomiting occurs when peristaltic motion of the muscles in the oesophagus and stomach is reversed under orders from the vomiting centre in the brain. That centre can be stimulated by direct nervous signals from the gut and probably by a hormone or hormones in the blood, but vomiting can also be caused by disturbances of the visual and balance centres in the brain better known as motion sickness.

DILL
(*Anethum graveolens*) A tall, single-stalked annual with long, feathery leaves that droop, and an unpleasant smell. Sometimes it is mistaken for FENNEL which grows taller and has less smell.

Dill is a seasoning often used in brine to make salt or dill pickles out of CUCUMBERS. As with most native herbs, there are many claims for its efficacy as a cure, for example, of wind, hiccough and sores around the anus. For the latter, it is applied directly.

DISTILLATION
The process of converting a liquid to a gas, usually by heating, condensing the gas by cooling and collecting the condensed liquid, the distillate. SPIRITS are distillations from fermented CARBOHYDRATES; for example, whisky and gin are distilled from FERMENTATION of cereals. The spirituous distillate consists almost entirely of ALCOHOL and WATER to which flavouring and COLOUR may be added.

Distilled water is purified of minerals and bacteria, and it also loses those electrical properties that cause water to fur up steam irons.

DIVERTICULITIS
A disease characterized by infection and inflammation of small pockets (diverticula; sing.: diverticulum) in the wall of the large intestine. Diverticulitis is common in older people. In the west, it occurs even in the middle-aged. Symptoms are constipation interrupted by occasional diarrhoea, mild abdominal pain and sometimes bleeding from the rectum. The bleeding cannot be distinguished from that caused by piles, but piles can usually be easily felt by inserting a finger into the anus.

Diverticulitis arises because faeces get stuck in the pockets. Until the mid-1970s, the most common treatment was a bland, easily-absorbed, soft diet; for example, white

BREAD, well-cooked VEGETABLES and as little FAT as possible. The idea was to reduce the amount of waste in the bowel. Because of the acceptance of FIBRE as an important dietary constituent, that treatment has now been much modified. Although fats may still be discouraged, more roughage is usually recommended. Even in the aged, the disease shows improvement more consistently with a high-fibre diet. Many doctors now suggest BRAN not just as a treatment but also as a preventive. Severe diverticulitis was treated surgically by removal of the infected section of the intestinal wall, but this measure is now rare.

DUROMINE ℞

A drug given in the form of pills to suppress appetite. It is available only on a doctor's prescription.

Duromine is a synthetic chemical, phentermine. It works by inhibiting the brain centre which regulates the desire for food. Like other brain-acting stimulants (see APISATE, TENUATE, TERONAC), Duromine may become addictive. It can also cause depression, agitation, insomnia, stomach upset, dizziness, tremor, headache, chills and possibly psychotic episodes. Perhaps of more concern, after a period of time that varies with the patient and the dose, the drug loses its effectiveness.

Another name for the same drug is Ionamin.

DUROPHET ℞

A drug given in the form of pills to suppress appetite. It is available only on a doctor's prescription.

Because it is an amphetamine and addictive, Durophet is infrequently prescribed today. Other side-effects also occur. Amphetamine is a stimulant that acts in the brain. See also FILON.

E

EGG
1. The ovum; a spheroidal object produced by the female containing the germ of a new individual within a membrane, shell or both. 2. A food, perhaps the most universally used and one of the most versatile from the standpoint of preparation.

In the west, almost the only eggs eaten are laid by the domestic hen. Duck, goose and turkey eggs are occasionally eaten, and such delicacies as plovers' eggs and caviar (fish eggs) have their special markets. All birds' eggs have essentially the same structure and contain similar NUTRIENTS. Duck eggs have somewhat more fat than chicken eggs. The intensity of yolk colour is due to a pigment in grasses, but the pigment has no nutritional value, and the colour gives no indication of quality or freshness. Raw free-range eggs may contain more of the VITAMINS, folic acid and B_{12}, but otherwise they have no greater nutritional value than battery eggs providing the battery hens have been fed with a balanced 'natural' diet. Battery eggs can be just as fresh as free-range. Nor apart from their colour is there a distinction between brown and white eggs except that the former are laid by brown hens and the latter, by white.

Eggs are easily digested and the nutrients easily absorbed providing the egg is cooked. In raw eggs, one of the protein components of the egg white, avidin, can combine with a vitamin, biotin, and with IRON, preventing their ABSORPTION. The notion that eggs cause constipation is a misapprehension which may have arisen because there is so little waste residue from eating them.

Hard-boiled eggs are just as digestible as those cooked in other ways. The green ring sometimes seen around the yolk of a hard-boiled egg is caused by a reaction between iron in the yolk and a chemical, sulphide, released by the protein in egg white as it coagulates during cooking. The ring can be prevented by boiling for the shortest possible time, about ten minutes, and quickly cooling in cold WATER. Old eggs in which the protein has begun to break down are more likely to develop green rings when they are hard-boiled than fresh eggs.

As the egg ages, various changes take place short of decomposition. Water moves from the white to the yolk causing the normally round yolk to flatten. The white becomes thinner and more runny. The air space increases, partly because a gas, carbon dioxide, forms in the egg though most of it escapes through the porous shell. Eventually, the yolk breaks and the proteins break down causing formation of hydrogen sulphide, a gas that gives the characteristic smell of rotten eggs. Because the smell is so objectionable, food poisoning from bad eggs is rare. On the other hand, bacteria and viruses can enter cracked eggs. Although their growth is inhibited by the alkaline environment (see BASE) produced by the egg protein, these organisms may cause disease if the egg is eaten.

Eggs are a valuable source of nutrients, with important exceptions: vitamin C is missing completely, and there is virtually no CARBOHYDRATE. Eggs have the highest CHOLESTEROL content of any common food excepting dairy products and offal. The table shows the nutrients in 100g or roughly two size 5 eggs:

	Raw	Boiled	Fried	Poached	Omelette (incl. butter)	Scrambled (incl. milk, butter)
Calories	147	147	232	155	190	246
Fat (g, all in yolk)	10.9	10.9	19.5	11.7	16.4	22.7
Cholesterol (mg, yolk)	450	450	*	480	410	410
Protein (g)	12.3	12.3	14.1	12.4	10.6	10.5
Potassium (mg)	140	140	180	120	120	130
Calcium (mg)	52	52	64	52	47	60
Phosphorus (mg)	220	220	260	240	190	190
Vitamins:						
A (microg, yolk)	140	140	140	140	190	130
B_1 (mg)[†]	0.09	0.08	0.07	0.07	0.07	0.07
B_2 (mg)	0.47	0.45	0.42	0.38	0.32	0.33
B_3 (mg)	3.68	3.68	4.21	3.72	3.17	3.12
B_6 (mg)	0.11	0.10	0.09	0.09	0.08	0.08

Tables continues on next page.

	Raw	Boiled	Fried	Poached	Omelette (incl. butter)	Scrambled (incl. milk, butter)
Vitamins: (Continued)						
Folic acid (microg)**	25	22	17	16	15	15
B_{12} (microg)**	1.7	1.7	1.7	1.7	1.5	1.4
Biotin (mg)	25	25	25	25	22	20
D (microg, yolk)†	1.75	1.75	1.75	1.75	1.57	1.54
E (mg)	1.6	1.6	1.6	1.6	1.5	1.6

* Depends on fat used for frying.
† Values may be higher if hen is fed a supplement.
** Values are for battery eggs. Free-range eggs are higher.

EMULSIFIER

A food ADDITIVE used to form a stable mixture between two substances which do not otherwise mix. One familiar example is the EGG yolk in mayonnaise. Mayonnaise consists basically of OIL and VINEGAR, but vinegar which is mostly WATER will not mix with oil. If the two liquids are stirred or shaken together, the oil will break up into droplets in the vinegar, and when the temporary emulsion is allowed to stand, the two constituents separate and the oil floats to the surface. Egg yolk contains chemicals called lipoproteins, a LIPID linked to a PROTEIN (see LOW-DENSITY LIPOPRO-TEIN), which act as emulsifiers. Thus, in making mayonnaise the oil is slowly whipped into the egg yolk, and the vinegar is added just as slowly to form the familiar thick, yellowish dressing which lasts more or less indefinitely under refrigeration.

Emulsifiers are used in BREAD, MARGARINE, chocolate and other confectionery as well as in SOFT DRINKS where they help to mix air and water in the form of bubbles. Newer CONVENIENCE FOODS which depend on emulsifiers to make them palatable include SOUP powder, instant potatoes and puddings, COFFEE whiteners and powdered drinks. Emulsifiers retain air inside FAT globules reducing ice-crystal formation in ice-cream. In homemade ice-cream, egg yolks are again the best emulsifiers.

Emulsifiers consist of molecules with two parts: one dissolves in water and the other in fat. The technical name for such molecules is 'amphipathic'. In egg yolk, the amphipathic molecules are the lipoproteins, the lipid portion being soluble in fat, and the protein in water.

Commercial emulsifiers are also often natural substances such as LECITHIN. Others are mixtures of natural and synthetic substances, for example, triglycerides (see LIPID) with a new compound, polyoxyethelene sorbitan, based on the natural ALCOHOL, sorbitol. One emulsifier, quillaia, is an extract of a South American tree bark.

Fifty-seven emulsifiers are permitted in the UK plus two that are tin-greasing compounds. Because the law requires that no new compound be authorized if one already on the list does the same job, each one of the emulsifiers is designed to serve a specific purpose. For example, quillaia produces a head of foam in soft drinks because it contains saponin, akin to soap in its ability to foam though not in anything else. Lecithins are the main permitted emulsifiers for CHEESE products. Modified triglycerides combined with weak organic ACIDS such as acetic, lactic and citric are used in bread-making. The best emulsifier for a product is a matter of judgement based on experience and a knowledge of chemistry.

Many emulsifiers are also STABILIZERS. Examples are those commonly used in bread-making.

ENERGEN ®
A food consisting of starch-reduced wheat crispbread with added BRAN. Each slice contains 18 CALORIES, 2g of PROTEIN, 1.9g of CARBOHYDRATE and 0.4g of FAT. The BREAD is made from wheat gluten, MALT, SALT, VEGETABLE fat, wheat bran, YEAST, caramel for colouring and a flavouring. (See SLIMMING AID.)

ENERGY
In general, the capacity for doing work. In biology, the capacity for maintaining life including growth and reproduction. So defined, energy is the reason for eating (leaving aside the social aspects of food consumption).

With a few exceptions such as black COFFEE, black TEA

and WATER, all food is a source of energy. With the exceptions noted, all foods contribute CALORIES, a measurement of the energy content of food. The major NUTRIENTS, CARBOHYDRATES, FATS and PROTEINS, can all be converted to energy, though at different rates. Thus, the same weight of carbohydrate and protein provide about the same energy, but an equivalent weight of fat supplies more than twice as much.

MINERALS and VITAMINS do not contribute to energy directly, but a person eating a high-energy diet of pure fat would starve without them. This is because energy-producing chemical changes cannot take place without minerals and vitamins. Two examples out of the thousands afforded by our bodies will make the point clear.

The most familiar role played by a mineral may be that of IRON in haemoglobin. The iron atom actually carries the oxygen we breathe in to our tissues. Obviously, without red blood corpuscles – they are red because they contain haemoglobin – most chemical reactions including those producing energy would cease. That is, the person would die of anoxia, oxygen insufficiency.

As to vitamins, vitamin B_3 prevents the symptoms of a disease called pellagra. Symptoms include skin sores, diarrhoea, a swollen tongue and severe mental disturbances. Eventually, without the vitamin the patient dies because the cells are unable to convert food to energy. Vitamin B_3 is a constituent of a coenzyme, that is, a factor required by an ENZYME. Enzymes which cannot function without this vitamin-based coenzyme play a direct role in the chemical changes that produce cellular energy.

The food we eat is not converted directly to energy. It must undergo complicated processing first. Many of the steps also require energy. In broad outline, conversion of food to energy begins with the DIGESTIVE PROCESS and the ABSORPTION of simple SUGARS and other nutrients. With the exception of lactic acid which is only important for short periods after intense manual labour or EXERCISE, the basic source of energy is the sugar, glucose. Energy from other carbohydrates, fat and protein can be released only if these substances are first converted to glucose. This simple molecule is broken down into its constituent elements, carbon, hydrogen and oxygen, which are recombined at the end of the energy-producing transformation as carbon dioxide and water. Ultimately, the energy that was stored in glucose came from sunlight inasmuch as plants synthesize carbohydrates out of water and carbon dioxide using the energy of the sun.

Note that although fats and proteins can be used to supply energy, they also perform other vital functions in the body. Food proteins supply the AMINO ACIDS from which new protein is synthesized for growth and repair. Food fat also plays many roles, for example, as the raw material for the white sheaths that cover and protect nerves. Even carbohydrates perform functions other than energy production. Sugars contribute to cell-to-cell communication. Every one of these functions depends on biosynthetic processing by body cells, and biosynthesis cannot occur without energy.

Although it is possible to work out average energy requirements for men and women of different ages and occupations (see Appendix I), very few of us conform to an average. Needs vary even from day to day. Holidays may seem to be a time for rest and relaxation, for example, but driving, swimming and dancing absorb a lot more energy than sitting at a desk. The following table shows the Calories per minute used up by men and women engaged in the specified activities:

Activity	Men	Women
Sleeping	4.5	3.8
Sitting quietly	5.8	4.8
Cooking	8.8	7.1
Polishing a table	18	14.6
Walking at 3mph	15.5	12.6
Office work	7.5	6.7
Lorry driving	6.7	not available
Work in commercial laundry, garage	17.2	13.4
Golfing, sailing	10.5–21	8.3–16.5
Dancing, tennis	21–31.5	16.5–25
Athletics, football	31.5+	25+

Given these wide variations, the best rule is that the ideal food intake for a healthy adult should contain energy equal to the requirements for the day. Pregnant women, children and adults recovering from serious illness need both more energy and more protein. The more we sit about, on the other hand, the less we ought to eat – a truism that too many people forget too often.

Whether it comes from carbohydrate, fat or protein, excess energy intake will be stored for future use either as GLYCOGEN or as body fat. Unfortunately, the body cannot rid itself of excess energy like it can excrete excess water by increasing its urine output. This is a biological fact of some interest, not only to those struggling to lose weight. It may reflect a positive adaptation to an environment which is unpredictably hostile; for example, a hunter can never be sure when he might become the hunted. In such a situation, he would need all the energy he could find without stopping for a meal. Whatever the reason for the body's determination to conserve every Calorie of unused energy (and it must be said that physiologists steer clear of such a question), dieters know the effort needed to reduce those stores. Therefore, the kind of diet depends on individual taste providing that it includes adequate nutrients. Here is a partial list of foods organized into energy groups from high to low:

Calories per ounce	Food
185–235	Cooking fats, oils, butter, margarine, cream cheese
85–160	Biscuits, cakes, dry CEREALS, NUTS, sugar, CHEESE, fat MEAT (e.g. bacon), double cream, chocolate, dried whole MILK
35–85	Lean meat, fatty FISH (e.g. mackerel), EGGS, BREAD, single cream
35 and under	White fish, most fresh FRUIT, fresh VEGETABLES, whole milk

If we take the figure of 2200 Calories per day as ideal for the average healthy woman aged eighteen to fifty-four who is not pregnant (see Appendix I), the list above shows that a well-balanced diet can be immensely flexible. Here, for example, is a menu for a day:

Breakfast, about 280 Calories	juice of 1 orange 1 slice wholemeal toast with ½oz butter or margarine black tea or coffee
Lunch, about 700 Calories	2 boiled eggs 1 slice wholemeal bread with ½oz butter or margarine 1 small glass of milk 1 small chocolate
Dinner, about 1200 Calories	6oz white fish, grilled with ½oz butter or margarine 6 brussels sprouts, boiled 2 new potatoes, boiled 1 medium carrot, boiled or raw 1 glass white wine 1 tangerine 1oz Cheddar cheese and 2 cream crackers

Total Calories: 2180

Using any Calorie table or the entries in this book, you can work out your own food combinations almost infinitely. Note that each of the three sample meals above contains adequate minerals, vitamins and FIBRE. The luncheon chocolate and the dinner glass of wine are pure indulgences providing almost no nutritional value except energy, but they illustrate how easy it is to control your energy intake without reducing the quality, variety and pleasure of eating.

ENZYME
A PROTEIN with the function of a catalyst: that is, it facilitates a chemical change that would take place more slowly without it. The enzyme itself emerges unchanged from the chemical process it catalyses and is indefinitely available for reuse.

Our bodies contain thousands of enzymes, not all of

which have yet been identified. Indeed, the first enzymes to be observed are among those that act during the DIGESTIVE PROCESS. Examples include amylase and pepsin. Most enzymes function inside body cells. They speed up chemical changes which would otherwise take place far too slowly to support life in the prevailing body conditions of temperature and ACID-base balance (see BASE). A good example may be seen in the breakdown of glucose to provide ENERGY. Dozens of enzymes play a role in this process. Without them, an organism endangered by a predator would simply be unable to summon up the energy needed to escape. In short, enzymes are an absolute prerequisite for life.

Each enzyme consists of a protein molecule; that is, it is a long chain of AMINO ACIDS. (Some enzymes are actually two or more proteins, but their structural characteristics are similar.) Atomic forces within and between the amino acids cause the whole molecule to roll up like a rubber band rubbed between the hands. Since each enzyme consists of a different sequence of amino acids, it follows that each enzyme has a different shape and form. The enzyme's distinctive form precisely determines its function because each of the thousands of enzymes performs only one catalytic act; it facilitates only one chemical change. The change may entail breaking down another chemical, known as the enzyme's substrate, and the break will always occur between the same two atoms in the substrate. Or the change may be the removal of oxygen or hydrogen (see OXIDATION) from the substrate, or joining two molecules (i.e. two substrates) together. One enzyme probably acts only on one kind of chemical. Thus, those that break down LIPIDS are called lipases. Those that break down proteins are called proteinases; CARBOHYDRATES, carbohydrases. The point is that because it has a distinctive shape, each molecular ball of linked amino acids performs a distinctive function. The reason for this is that in the process of rolling itself up, two or more amino acids from different parts of the chain are brought close together to form an active site. When a substrate enters the active site, atomic forces between the juxtaposed amino acids cause the typical chemical change. Once the substrate has been changed – for example, joined or split – the altered atomic forces cause the active site to release the substrate, and the enzyme is ready for action again. The enzyme is a chemical machine designed specifically to couple together or split apart two atoms.

The last important characteristic of enzymes for our purposes is their origin. How do we obtain our supply of these vital molecules? We inherit them, not directly but in the form of genes. Each of the thousands of genes that make up the forty-six chromosomes (twenty-three from each parent) in most of our body cells may specify the synthesis by the cell of an enzyme. All genes probably direct the synthesis of a protein, but not all proteins are enzymes. Nor do all cells have the same complement of enzymes despite the fact that they all have the same genes. How one cell contains one set of enzymes and another cell, another set is by no means clear, but the fact that they do explains why some cells are nerve cells and some cells in the intestinal wall absorb NUTRIENTS. Furthermore, the colour of our eyes, our height, our sex and most of our other features are basically determined by our genes which specify our unique blend of proteins, including enzymes. Thus, whereas most white British adults can digest whole MILK, a minority of Indian adults cannot. They have lost the ability to synthesize enough lactase, an enzyme required for efficient digestion of milk. This is a normal condition and not a disease but, in every country, there are some infants born without an enzyme to break down the amino acid, PHENYLALANINE. If they are not fed a carefully controlled diet, they will develop the symptoms of a disease called phenylketonuria. There are other digestive disorders that reflect short-term disruption of an enzyme supply, but these are not diseases originating in the genes and are usually amenable to control or cure. For example, 'dyspepsia' may reflect a temporary failure of pepsin production by cells in the stomach wall brought on by an excess of acidic food. The cure may be a teaspoonful of bicarbonate of soda in half a glass of water. On the other hand, genetic errors can produce serious and lasting diseases because an enzyme is permanently missing or malformed.

In terms of diet and nutrition, enzymes are important not only in the digestive process but also in commercial food PROCESSING and as food ADDITIVES. Both uses of enzymes have ancient antecedents. Perhaps the oldest application of enzymes to food occurs in FERMENTATION, a chemical change catalysed by enzymes in YEAST and certain bacteria. Making leavened BREAD, CHEESE and YOGHURT all depend on enzymic action. Even meat TENDERIZERS have a long history. Note that enzymes used in processing cannot contribute directly to our own digestive process. For example, eating yeast does not cause alcoholic fermentation in the stomach. This is because enzymes themselves are proteins; any we eat are rapidly broken down by our own stomach enzymes and hydrochloric acid. Incidentally, it is because they are proteins that enzymes cannot be given as pills to replace any that are missing or malfunctioning. Nor can they be injected because the immune defences attack and destroy foreign protein (SEE ALLERGY, FOOD), though genetic engineering may make it possible to grow bacteria that can make human enzymes.

Enzymes are added to food products for many reasons. For example, MEAT scraps and FISH waste contain valuable protein, but are 'unattractive' foods. By adding pepsin and another digestive enzyme, trypsin, however, they can be hydrolysed and processed to form acceptable products. Because the protein is already partially digested, these hydrolysates are especially useful as food for people who are recovering from periods of starvation. Enzymes are also used to degrease bones and to clean shellfish as well as to tenderize ordinary cuts of meat. Glucose oxidase, an enzyme obtained commercially from a mould, *Aspergillus niger*, will prevent browning in dried eggs, meats and dehydrated potatoes. Glucose oxidase removes oxygen and has been used to stabilize (SEE STABILIZER) citrus-fruit-based SOFT DRINKS, to prevent rancidity in butter and BEER and the vinegarization of WINE. Peroxidase from the same mould, *Aspergillus niger*, or from a bacterium, *Micrococcus lysodeiktikus*, is used in cheese-making, stabilization of milk-souring cultures such as yoghurt and to pasteurize EGGS. Carbohydrases including amylase may also be obtained from bacteria. They are used in baking to break down complex SUGARS so that they are more easily digested and to make stabilizers and EMULSIFIERS.

Enzymes are not directly covered by regulations controlling food additives. Those obtained from animal and plant tissue normally used for food, from micro-organisms found in food or used in its preparation (as in yoghurt, for example) are considered safe by the FAO/WHO Expert Committee on Food Additives. Enzymes from other micro-organisms, for example, disease-causing bacteria, are subject to special testing like any other food additives. In the UK at the end of 1984, use of enzymes is regulated by the FAO/WHO and EEC recommendations and by the provisions of the 1955 Food and Drugs Act which prohibits the use of unsafe additives in food.

EPSOM SALTS
The most familiar of the saline laxatives, laxatives which act by retaining WATER in the intestines thus increasing both the fluid content and the speed of movement of wastes. Chemically, epsom salts are magnesium sulphate.

Epsom salts act rapidly, usually within two hours, if taken before breakfast with a glass of warm water. They increase osmotic pressure into the intestine, retaining water and drawing water from the body under some circumstances. It is this potential dehydration effect of the saline laxatives that explains the need to take them well-diluted.

Other magnesium compounds used as laxatives in the UK are magnesium carbonate and magnesium hydroxide. In Britain, saline laxatives made of sodium phosphate may be used as enemas but not taken orally.

See also BRAN, CELEVAC, PREFIL.

EXERCISE
Activity, any activity that gets you out of a chair and away from the television, but preferably an activity that gets you

out of the house into the open air. Exercise is as important to health and fitness as good nutrition through a CALORIE-controlled diet.

There are four major fallacies about exercise, each related to the others.

1. Anyone can benefit from exercise. Medical authorities consider this statement to be true for many people, but perhaps not for most people. As the population ages, more of us are over thirty-five than under. Any reputable statement recommending exercise must begin with the warning: *if you are over thirty-five, consult your doctor before embarking on any new or different exercise regimen.* If you are fifty and have been doing housework every day for thirty years, then climbing stairs and hoovering are not going to endanger your health. But running for thirty minutes in the morning before you begin the day's chores might. Ask your doctor. (In any case, you should begin with a five-minute slow run and gradually increase both your time and your speed.) Even people under thirty-five must consult a doctor before beginning any new exercise if they have heart trouble or breathing problems such as bronchitis or asthma. This is especially the case for diabetics for whom exercise is nevertheless important (see DIABETES).

2. You have to walk an enormous distance to lose any weight. This idea grew up because ENERGY expenditure was calculated ultra-scientifically as the amount of oxygen used to perform different tasks, a measurable and fairly consistent quantity. It is still a valid indicator of energy consumption, but it must be adjusted to take into consideration the knock-on effect of exercise in two respects: the energy required to replace tissues, for example, PROTEIN in muscles that has been used up during exercise, and the fact that energy used during exercise is cumulative. That is, if you walk at a normal speed of about 4mph for thirty minutes every day, you will use up Calories equal to just over 20lb of FAT in a year. By increasing the length of your walk to about thirty-seven minutes or the speed to about five miles per hour, you almost double the energy expenditure to the equivalent of more than 35lb of body fat lost in

a year. The calculation is independent of what you eat, but of course you can put back the weight by eating an extra 200 Calories a day. Which brings us to the third common fallacy about exercise.

3. It makes you so hungry that you eat that much more. Just think about this statement: you normally eat to make it possible for you to perform the daily round. For many people, that includes two miles of walking (half an hour at 4mph). It is simply not true that if you were to walk another two miles, you would eat another 200 Calories: four slices of ordinary white BREAD or two tablespoons of butter.

4. Finally, it is said that overweight and obese people do not lose weight if they exercise. In fact, there is some truth in this. The amount of body fat depends in part on the number of fat cells in the body. The number of fat cells is determined by three factors: inheritance, the amount of fat on the body during childhood and, possibly, food intake during adult life. The relative influence of each of these factors is poorly understood, but the more fat cells in the body, the harder it is to lose fat. For this reason, exercise alone may not significantly influence the weight of obese people. On the other hand, the psychological aspects of OBESITY also play a role. To the degree that overweight stems from compulsive eating, exercise may serve as an excuse for more of the same behaviour. See also, the previous fallacy. But at the very least, the exercise helps to tone the body and improve the circulation, and it may also lose some pounds.

Regardless of body size, exercise tends to redistribute body tissue. A study of normal young people shows that actual weight remains about the same after exercise, but the amount of body fat declines and inches disappear from waists and thighs. At an American women's college, students doing forty minutes of dancing per day three days a week for ten weeks lost no weight. Yet many of the students reported that their clothes were becoming loose. What had happened in both studies was the same: muscle had replaced fat. Fat takes up much more space than the same weight of muscle, so their bodies became slimmer.

Having examined the objections, we can now look at the demonstrable advantages of regular exercise within the capacity of the individual.

1. Exercise tones the body keeping muscles in condition and relatively reducing body fat.

2. Exercise increases muscle strength. Use reduces flabbiness by adding to the number and size of muscle cells. (See comments on fat cells in fallacy 4, above.)

3. Exercise increases joint flexibility, reducing and delaying the impact of degenerative joint diseases such as rheumatism and of common complaints like low-back pain.

4. Exercise improves circulation of the blood because it strengthens the muscles in blood vessels and in the heart as well as the leg muscles which contribute greatly to the efficient return of blood to the heart through the long veins in the legs. The general improvement in circulation may reduce the incidence of two common diseases, high blood pressure without any discernible cause and strokes, accidental blockages of blood vessels in the brain that cause damage to brain cells.

The number of Calories you use up during exercise depends in part on your weight. For example, a rat uses about 3 per cent of its daily energy output by running or walking six miles a day. A person walking the same distance uses 10 per cent of his total energy output, and an elephant uses more than 20 per cent. As a rough guide, you may estimate that for any given exercise, you will expend 10 per cent more energy per 15lb of weight over 150lb, and 10 per cent less per 15lb of weight under 150lb.

Although the kind of exercise you do must fit your physical capacity, your time and inclination also determine your choice. Not everyone enjoys games or gymnastics, but few people really dislike swimming, bicycling, running or a good walk. Even dancing, which uses 4–6 Calories per minute in a ballroom and 7–9 at a disco for a person weighing 150lb, gardening using 8–9 Calories a minute and sexual intercourse – 4–6 Calories – provide useful exercise. Whatever you choose to do, do some exercise, do it regularly and begin slowly to build up your endurance.

Despite the caveat about exercise for people over thirty-five, age should be no bar to fitness for normally healthy people. Providing your doctor approves, moreover, there is no form of exercise from which the over-sixties are debarred. More than one sixty-year-old has run the London Marathon and not been the last to finish. You must simply trim your cloth to suit you. Fast walking may have to replace running, at least for part of the course. Tennis doubles are a little less demanding than singles, and for most older people, golf is more appropriate than push-ups. Though muscles are no longer as strong nor joints as flexible when we grow older, ageing is no excuse for sluggishness, even less for obesity.

Most authorities still consider jogging the best all-round exercise. There has been a lot of publicity in the early 1980s about deaths while jogging, but none of those who died is known to have consulted a doctor before starting. A person weighing 150lb who jogs at a rate of 5mph will use up about 11 Calories per minute. Benefits in muscle tone and blood circulation are no greater than from cycling or swimming both of which produce roughly the same Calorie consumption. In swimming, different muscles are being used. Cycling, swimming and many other more special forms of exercise require equipment, however, whereas all you need to jog is a good pair of running shoes. Jogging and walking can be done anywhere, at any time and in any weather.

The following table shows some activities with the approximate Calorie expenditure per minute for a person weighing 150lb. Add 10 per cent for every 15 lb of weight over 150lb and subtract 10 per cent for every 15lb under 150lb. Variations will also occur because of the skill and vigour with which you perform, but such variations are impossible to calculate. Bear in mind that one slice of white bread contains about 50 Calories.

Activity	Calories per minute
Backpacking	6–14
Badminton	5–11
Bowling	5–6
Calisthenics	5
Cycling (5–15 mph)	5–12
Carpentry	3–9
Dancing, ballroom	4–6
disco	7–9
DIY (painting, plumbing)	4–5
Driving	3
Farming (ploughing with horse)	6–7
Fishing, from bank or boat	3–5
wading	7–8
Gardening (digging etc.)	8–9
Golf (walking and carrying bag)	3–6
Handball	8–12
Horseshoe pitching	4
Heavy housework (e.g. scrubbing)	5–6
Ironing	4
Jogging	6.5–12.5
Motor cycling	3–5
Ping-pong	5–9
Pool, billiards	2
Sailing	3–7
Sitting	1.5
Skating (ice or roller)	5–15
Skipping	8–11
Soccer	8–12
Squash	8–12
Standing	2–3
Swimming, backstroke	6–12.5
breast stroke	6–12.5
butterfly	14
crawl	6–12
sidestroke	11
Tennis	7–12
Walking	6–8

F

FAO

Food and Agriculture Organization. One of the special-purpose organizations of the United Nations, with its headquarters in Rome. The FAO develops agricultural policies, particularly for the newly-emergent nations, supplies guidance on a range of subjects from crop rotation to soil improvement, examines and reports on machinery, food PROCESSING and food ADDITIVES, the latter with the WHO. Members are countries which must also be members of the UN, though UN membership does not automatically confer FAO membership.

FAT

With CARBOHYDRATE and PROTEIN one of the major NUTRI-ENTS. In food at room temperature, fat is either solid as in MEAT and CHEESE or liquid as in OIL. It is, of course, easy to liquiefy solid fat with heat but less easy to solidify oils at temperatures available in the ordinary kitchen. The separated fats in butter, lard and cream have very low melting points.

A more important distinction is between the saturated animal fats and the unsaturated VEGETABLE fats. The latter are believed to be better for us because they are less likely to fur up blood vessels than animal fats. Vegetable fats also contribute linoleic acid, the one essential fat constituent that the body cannot synthesize. The details of chemical structure and of the chemical differences between saturated and unsaturated fats are dealt with in the entry on LIPID. In keeping with British practice, the present entry deals with fat as a constituent of the diet.

Apart from the separated fats, the best food sources in descending order of their fat content are peanuts, streaky bacon, chocolate, Cheddar cheese, pork loin, plain biscuits, herring, roast beef and EGGS. Vegetables with the exception of some beans, and FRUIT with the exception of bananas contain almost no fat. TEA and COFFEE without milk are fat-free.

Fat provides more ENERGY per unit weight than either carbohydrates or protein, 9 CALORIES per gram as against about 4 Calories for each of the other two. Thus, fat is the most valuable and the most expensive source of energy. Most people would agree that it is also the most delicious, even including SUGAR. Were it otherwise, the dangers from excessive fat consumption would presumably be less

apparent. Heart and circulatory diseases are far more frequent in countries such as the UK and the US where
dietary fat provides something like 40 per cent of our
energy intake than in countries such as Japan where the
percentage is much lower. All authorities now agree that
we should reduce our dietary fat to no more than 35 per
cent of energy intake as quickly as possible (see DIET,
BALANCED). In practice, this means eating leaner cuts of
meat, less fatty FISH (plaice, for example, instead of herring
or mackerel), fewer fried foods, skimmed rather than
whole MILK, less butter and cream. Fat-reduced diets are
recommended for most adults. Though fat reduction may
be less important for growing children, the intake must
still be controlled. In Britain, eight-year-olds have been
diagnosed with serious arterial disease, possibly related to
their over-dependence on deep-fried fish and chips.
Reduced-fat diets will of course supply ample energy, but
they are usually more bulky; that is, they contain more
food weight-for-weight.

Bulkier diets probably contribute a bonus, moreover:
they move more rapidly through the intestines probably
reducing flatulence, heartburn and more serious digestive
disorders such as DIVERTICULITIS (see also FIBRE). Fat
moves out of the stomach more slowly than other nutrients
because it is emulsified but only partially broken down by
gastric juice (see BILE and DIGESTIVE PROCESS). However,
unless your doctor prescribes it for you, a completely fat-
free diet is unwise for two reasons: four VITAMINS, A, D, E
and K, are dissolved in fat and must be taken as drug
supplements if they are not obtained from dietary fat.
(Vitamin D is also produced in the skin by sunshine, but
in northern climates, dietary vitamin intake is essential.)
Second, fat ABSORPTION also assists absorption of two B
vitamins, folic acid and B_{12}. It is well to remember that fat
can be eaten pure, as in cream, whereas WATER or heat are
needed to make most carbohydrate and protein edible.
Exceptions like sugar spring to mind, but any cook recognizes that meat, vegetables and cereals take expensive time

FAT   93

and energy to prepare. Energy-rich fats may be expensive
to produce but not to prepare.

The body can synthesize fat from carbohydrate and
protein. This fact raises problems for people on fat-free
diets. For example, it is not hard to cut down the amount
of CHOLESTEROL in what we eat, and cholesterol is a fat
often associated with circulatory diseases. The blood levels
of cholesterol are not necessarily related directly to dietary
intake, however, in part because we synthesize our own
cholesterol in the liver. In theory, each of us has a balancing
mechanism which sets both the amount of fat circulating in
our blood in the form of various fatty molecules and the
amount in the more visible fat layers that lie between skin
and muscles. The trouble is that this balancing mechanism
has not been identified. It seems to operate with great
differences in different but entirely normal people, quite
apart from sex differences in body shape. These variations
are controlled by the genes and the sex HORMONES. Some
people tend to carry more fat than others. There are two
possible explanations for this, but both are controversial
because the evidence is far from straightforward. They may
be summarized as the basal metabolic rate (BMR) and
brown fat deposits.

Each of us has a BMR (see METABOLISM). Basal means
base, and the base rate can be precisely measured when the
body is relaxed and resting but not asleep. It is usually
measured in terms of the amount of air inhaled. There is
an average basal metabolism expressed as 100 but not a
'normal' basal metabolism. That is, variations of 15 to 20
points up or down may still be normal. However, people
living in a state of chronic under-nutrition or near starvation
may show a fall in BMR of as much as 15 per cent with a
further fall recorded as the effects of tissue loss due to
dietary insufficiency become manifest. Oddly, and some
would say regrettably, the reverse does not apply. Overeat-
ing does not lead to a concomitant rise in BMR. It has
been supposed that the extra energy from excess food might
be lost through heat production, but this is by no means
certain. In any case, not even lean subjects respond to

over-feeding by a significant rise in BMR. Although theory holds that OBESITY reflects either a lower than normal BMR or a less responsive BMR, the facts seem to support the view that there is no consistent difference in BMR between lean and obese people.

The second possible explanation for obesity has to do with brown fat deposits. Animals and human infants have two kinds of fat in their bodies, white and brown. All fat tissues consist of cells in the same way that muscle cells make up muscles. White fat is made up of cells containing relatively few fat droplets whereas brown fat cells contain many more droplets, more fat within the single cell. In conditions where the body requires heat, brown fat deposits are released and consumed to produce heat energy, at least in animals. Again in animals, when excess food is eaten, brown fat deposits are mobilized for heat energy increasing energy loss and lowering body weight. The theory, there-fore, is that obese people lack brown fat, or that there is some failure in the breakdown of the brown fat deposits they have. Unfortunately, there is no firm evidence that humans have brown fat at all let alone that lean people have more or burn more than obese people.

FENNEL

(*Arethum faeniculum*) A tall annual plant which may also run wild near sea-coasts. It has beautiful, long, green leaves, small yellow flowers and thick white roots. The leaves have a spinachy taste but contain more CARBO-HYDRATE than spinach, most of it indigestible FIBRE. Fennel provides about 27 CALORIES per 100g (3½oz).

Traditionally, roots and seeds as well as leaves were used as a tonic. In particular, fennel was believed to improve digestion, evacuation and urination. WINE in which the seeds have been boiled was said to help snake bite and the sting of poisonous plants, perhaps more an effect of any remaining ALCOHOL than of the plant elixir itself.

FERMENTATION

A chemical change which produces ALCOHOL in the juices of plants. BEER, SPIRITS and WINE are all products of fermentation, but the process as well as the plants used vary from drink to drink.

Fermentation requires conversion of SUGAR and other CARBOHYDRATES to ethyl alcohol and carbon dioxide by the activity of ENZYMES from micro-organisms. YEASTS supply the enzymes for beer, and bacteria are usually the sources for those that produce wine. The fermentation process breaks down the sugar molecule, releasing energy in the form of heat. The process also provides the NUTRIENTS for the growth and multiplication of the micro-organisms.

The breakdown of protein by enzymes from micro-organisms is usually referred to as putrefaction and does not produce ethyl alcohol.

FIBRE, FOOD

Those parts of edible leaves, FRUIT, roots, seed, stems and flowers that are not digested. Fibre-like FISH and MEAT constituents – for example, gristle – are not food fibre because no matter how tough they seem, they can be fully digested. Fibre is also called roughage and bulk, or by the technical name, unavailable CARBOHYDRATE.

STARCH and SUGAR, like PROTEIN and FAT, are fully digested in the healthy gut. Other carbohydrates such as CELLULOSE and gums cannot be absorbed (see ABSORPTION) because humans lack the ENZYMES needed to break them down into small enough units. Many other animals can digest what to us is fibre: for example, cows, goats, dogs and cats can use much more of the plant than we can. Among the bacteria that normally inhabit our gut, especially those in the large intestine, there are several species that break down fibre. We also absorb some of their products as digested food. On the whole, however, unavailable carbohydrate passes through the intestines more or less unchanged.

Food fibre is not a NUTRIENT. Until the early 1970s, it was often considered to be unimportant if not harmful. BRAN as a laxative has always had its champions, but the indigestibility of fibre caused some authorities to look on bran as an irritant. High-fibre diets tend to reduce the absorption of protein and the nutrient carbohydrates, probably because fibre bulk causes digested food to move more quickly through the intestines. For all of these reasons, fibre was often removed from processed foods.

The average British diet now contains about 20g of fibre a day. Rural African communities consume anywhere from 50 to 120g a day. During World War II when BREAD in the UK was made from less refined flour, fibre consumption rose to as much as 40g a day. VEGETARIANS eat about 42g a day. Many of the diseases associated with technically advanced western societies do not occur with the same frequency among rural Africans or vegetarians, and may even have been less common in Britain during World War II. One reason could be that fibre increases the speed with which food moves through the gut.

The diseases and disorders include CANCER of the colon, constipation, DIVERTICULITIS, heart and circulatory disorders and OBESITY. Excepting constipation, the evidence that high-fibre diets reduce the incidence of any of these conditions is statistical only in the same way that a link between smoking and lung cancer is statistical. Physiological cause-and-effect relationships between a lack of fibre and the listed disorders, except constipation, is controversial at best. Yet the fact remains that more people eating low-fibre diets than those on high-fibre diets are afflicted by them.

The 1983 discussion paper published by the National Advisory Committee on Nutrition Education (see DIET, BALANCED) recommends an increase in average food fibre intake to 25g a day immediately. CEREAL fibre may be more useful than VEGETABLE or FRUIT fibre. The following list gives the amount of fibre in 100g (3½oz) of selected foods and shows how easy it is to eat 25g of fibre a day:

Food	g fibre per 100g food
Wholemeal flour	11
White flour	2.5
Almonds, fresh coconut	10–15
Brazil nuts, peanuts, walnuts, cobnuts, chestnuts	5–10

Food	g fibre per 100g food
Currants, dates, blackberries, stewed prunes, raspberries	7–8.5
Gooseberries, fresh figs, strawberries, apples,* apricots,*	
pears,* plums, oranges, stewed rhubarb	2–2.5
Tangerines, stewed cooking apples, cherries	1.5–2
Peaches,* pineapple, cantaloupe	1–1.5
Grapes,* yellow melon, grapefruit	0.5–1
Spinach, peas, baked beans	5–6.5
Brussels sprouts, broad beans, broccoli	4–5
Leeks, mustard and cress, spring greens	3.5–4
Watercress, runner beans, carrots	3–3.5
Swede, cabbage, cauliflower, boiled lentils, mushrooms,	
parsnips, beetroot	2.5–3
Salads	1.5–2
Potatoes, radishes	1–1.5
Marrow, cucumber*	0.5–1

* Skin, pips and/or stems removed.

FILON ®
A drug designed to suppress appetite. It is available on doctor's prescription only, and it is not recommended in the United Kingdom. Filon consists of two amphetamine-like chemicals, phenbutrazate and phenmetrazine, both of which may be addictive. It acts in the brain to suppress the desire to eat. See also DUROPHET.

FIRMING AGENT
A food ADDITIVE which preserves VEGETABLE textures and holds their WATER content. Firming agents are used primarily in the canning industry. Chemicals permitted for these purposes are ordinary SALT, various CALCIUM salts, calcium hydroxide and two aluminium salts. All firming agents permitted in the UK may also act in other additive roles as BUFFERS, EMULSIFIERS or PRESERVATIVES.

FISH AND SHELLFISH
One of the most valuable sources of NUTRIENTS both from the standpoint of cost and from that of food bulk. For example, 100g (3½oz) of baked cod, price about £1.20 per

pound, can be favourably compared to 100g of grilled lean rump steak, price about £2.50 per pound.

	Cod	Beef
CALORIES	96	218
PROTEIN (g)	21.4	27.3
Essential AMINO ACIDS (mg/g) methionine	180	170
lysine	610	570
tryptophan	70	80
FAT (g)	1.2	14.6
MINERALS (mg) CALCIUM	22	7
IRON	0.4	1.9
PHOSPHORUS	190	220
POTASSIUM	350	380

About 19 per cent of our VITAMIN D supplied by food comes from fatty fish (see below). Yet the average British diet includes more than seven times more MEAT than fish.

In the minds of many shoppers, three questions seem to hang above the fish stalls of Britain: How fresh is it? How can you get more taste from it? How do you prepare it?

Although most experts agree that fresh fish has more taste than frozen, the fact is that modern fast-freezing techniques greatly reduce the chance that you will be offered stale fish in the market. Still, many people think that compared to meat, fish is bland. Of course, tastes differ, but with a modest use of HERBS and spices, fish FLAVOURS can be both varied and subtle. You should also remember that meat needs much longer cooking than most fish, and fish almost always lacks the tendinous matter than makes meat tough and hard to chew. People who have lost their own teeth will find fish much easier to eat than meat. As to the question of preparation, any good cookbook will give you dozens of suggestions. Whether it is baked, boiled, fried or grilled, fish is done when the flesh turns from translucent to a milky white or pink and separates easily with a fork.

From the standpoint of food value, there are two kinds of fish: white and fatty. The former includes cod, haddock, halibut, plaice, sole and whiting. The fatty fish include eel, herring, mackerel, pilchards, salmon, sardines, trout, tuna and whitebait. Skate and dogfish or hake are classed as cartilaginous fish but also have relatively high fat contents.

Fatty fish contain more Calories than white fish. The fats are largely polyunsaturated like VEGETABLE fats, however, and probably better for you than meat fats. In addition to providing our richest food sources of vitamin D, the fatty fish are good sources of vitamins A, E and K.

Shellfish are either crustaceans (shrimp, prawns, crab, lobster) or molluscs (snails, mussels, oysters, clams, whelks, cockles, winkles). Shellfish contain almost twice the SALT found in fish, slightly more CARBOHYDRATE and about the same protein, fat and Calories. All shellfish contain more iron than other fish. Weight for weight, cockles, oysters and whelks have as much iron as beef.

Shellfish poisoning is less common than episodes of shellfish allergies (see ALLERGY, FOOD), but you must be careful when gathering shellfish yourself. Sewage contamination can occur. Some red plankton carry a POISON which is held in the flesh of molluscs that eat them. Shellfish sold by your fishmonger is almost certainly fresh and clean, but there are simple rules for identifying a suspicious individual. For example, if after soaking for an hour or so in fresh water, a mussel remains shut, it is probably best to throw it away. Any that have not opened after boiling, moreover, should also be avoided. Any good cookbook will be a mine of such information. Like fish, shellfish require relatively little cooking.

Fresh fish rarely causes poisoning because its taste and smell become objectionable if bacterial decay has set in. Smoked fish, especially smoked trout, must be refrigerated until it is served. Even so, it cannot be kept more than a few days. Fish can contain methyl mercury, a poison and the source of much bad publicity about toxic canned tuna from Japan during the 1970s. Fortunately the mercury content of fish caught in British waters is so low that on average, you would have to eat a pound of fish every day to exceed the adult danger level. Mercury poisoning from British fish is far less likely than lead poisoning from British air.

Fatty fish can be canned, but white fish is usually better preserved by freezing; its flesh discolours during the canning process. The oldest methods of preserving fish, salting and smoking, are also still in use. Some protein is lost in salting, but smoking actually increases the nutrient content. The exception is vitamin B_1, most of which is lost in both canning and smoking.

Fish products such as fish cakes, pastes and fish fingers may contain ADDITIVES such as COLOUR (for example, yellow in smoked kippers), EMULSIFIERS, flavours and PRESERVATIVES. Frozen fish fingers may also contain ANTIOXIDANTS in the batter. The content of fish fingers is not subject to specific legal control, but they usually consist of between 50 and 70 per cent fish. Legal requirements for fish content of other fish products are:

Product	percentage of fish
Fish cakes	35
Fish pastes and spreads	70
excepting those marked, 'requires grilling'	None
excepting those with one other main ingredient	80
Potted fish	95
Potted fish and butter (fish and butter combines)	96

FLAVOUR

1. Taste plus smell. 2. A food ADDITIVE intended to enhance taste and/or smell. Both natural and added flavours consist of chemicals, often the same ones.

It is almost impossible to assess the relative importance of taste and smell in a flavour. The taste buds on the tongue, inside the cheeks and at the back of the mouth are, of course, the organs of taste and are linked by nerve cells to the brain. Taste buds respond to four 'tastes': sweet, sour or ACID, bitter and SALT. There are two reasons for the great variety of tastes we recognize: combinations of responses by taste buds, possibly including responses from those in different parts of the mouth; and the effects of the sense of smell.

Smell originates in olfactory nerve endings in the roof of

FLAVOUR   101

the nose. Different nerve cells respond to different smells
such as acrid or smoky. Refined smells like baking bread
or brewing must be learned, but they are no less influential
in determining taste. In fact, smell is probably more
important than taste in promoting appetite and distinguish-
ing among foods. To a person with a bad cold, an apple
has pretty much the same flavour as an onion.

Any one natural flavour may be a mixture of up to fifty
chemical components. For example, the HERB peppermint
contains isoamyl alcohol, menthone, menthyl isovalerate,
3-methylbutyraldehyde and isovaleric acid, among others.
The manufacturer who wants to synthesize a well-rounded
peppermint flavour must know not only the ingredients
but their quantities and relative strength.

Flavour is added to processed food to enhance natural
flavour, to replace losses due to processing, especially
cooking, and to flavour synthetic foods from instant puddings to cheese and bacon crisps. Some 1500 flavourings
are used by the food industry. They fall into four main
groups: foods such as anchovies or soy sauce, HERBS and
spices, extracts and distillates such as vanilla extract and
ginger oil, and synthetics. With more than 1000 specified
chemicals, synthetics are by far the largest group. Because
of the large number of natural components needed to
synthesize a flavour, the safety of any synthetic flavour
depends on the safety of each component. It would be best
if every component had been tested separately and, because
of possible chemical interactions, in combinations. However, with so many constituents, such detailed testing is
well-nigh impossible. There is no UK list of permitted
flavours, but in 1976 the Food Additives and Contaminants
Committee of the Ministry of Agriculture, Fisheries and
Food reported on a preliminary classification of 1585
flavourings. The classes are: flavours derived directly from
food, natural components of these flavours, synthetic substances which experience and testing indicate are probably
safe, synthetic substances considered safe if amounts used
are restricted and, finally, a group of thirteen banned items.
They are all natural, but they may all be toxic:

Hepatica (*Anemone hepatica*)
Deadly nightshade (*Atropa belladonna*)
White bryony (*Bryonia diocia*), roots only
Mexican goosefoot (*Chenopodium ambrosioides*)
Lily of the valley (*Convalleria majalis*)
Mezereon (*Daphne mezereum*)
Male fern (*Dryopteris filix-mas*), rhizomes only
Heliotropium europaeum, leaves only
Jamaica dogwood (*Piscidia erythrina*), roots only
Polypody (*Polypodium vulgare*), rhizomes only
Pomegranate (*Punica granatum*), roots only
Slippery elm (*Ulmus fulva*), bark only
Squill (*Urginea scilla*), bulb only

However, even common natural flavours contain toxins
which should limit their usefulness. These include cou-
marin (proposed limit: 5 mg/kg of bodyweight or 10 mg/l
of alcoholic drinks) and caffeine (300 mg/kg of body
weight). Of the hundreds of herbs and spices, only about
fifty are used in cooking. The discovery of toxins in some
of these common food ingredients has caused the UK
authorities to recommend specific testing and subsequent
control of all herbs and spices used for flavouring.

FLUORINE
A chemical element related to CHLORINE and thus naturally
a gas. Very small quantities of fluoride, a SALT of fluorine,
are an important component of bones and teeth. Although
the amount present is about one part in 10,000, fluoride
stabilizes and hardens these tissues.

TEA is the most significant food source of fluoride in the
British diet, containing 0.2 to 0.5mg per cup. Sea FISH also
contain fluoride. The total daily dietary intake averages
between 0.6 and 1.8mg. Children tend to eat much less
because they eat less food and drink little tea. The relatively
smaller amounts available to children is significant because
fluoride helps to harden tooth enamel during the years
from birth to about the age of ten when the teeth are
forming. After ten, fluoride probably has little effect.

Although dental decay in children is not caused by fluoride deficiency (see SUGAR), the incidence is reduced by about half if children drink WATER containing about 1mg per million of fluoride. In other words, children who drink fluoridated water from birth have about half as many fillings, decayed or missing teeth as children who drink unfluoridated water.

Fluorine is by no means an unmixed blessing. About 2g per day, more than a thousand times the average daily intake, is poisonous. Adding as much as 1.5 parts per million to drinking water can cause some people's tooth enamel to become mottled. The mottling is unsightly but does not weaken the teeth or increase decay. In children over ten and adults, furthermore, there is no evidence that fluoride protects the teeth, but that may be due in part at least to the fact that the principal tooth problem in adult mouths is gum disease rather than caries.

Nevertheless, there is no evidence that fluoride added to drinking water in recommended quantities causes damage. Perhaps the strongest argument advanced by those who oppose water fluoridation is moral: no one, they say, should be required to take a drug against their will. To protect children's teeth, they suggest either use of fluorine pills or direct application of fluoride to teeth. Pills containing 1mg of fluoride are available, but they must be taken once a day from birth for ten years to obtain the effect given by fluoridated water. As to direct application, fluoridated toothpastes and mouthwashes unfortunately do not seem to work. On the other hand, American and Soviet experiments with painting fluoride on the teeth have had promising results. The treatment is not available on the National Health Service, nor can there be any doubt that from the standpoint of cost effectiveness, fluoridated drinking water is the best protection against tooth decay in children.

F-PLAN DIET

A high-fibre, low-calorie diet based on the book, *The F-Plan*, by Audrey Eyton (1982). CALORIE reduction is achieved by reducing CARBOHYDRATES and FATS; for example, low-calorie salad dressings and calorie-free drinks (COFFEE, mineral WATER, TEA) or drinks with negligible calorie content (Diet Pepsi, Tab, Slimline) but not FRUIT juices because they contain all the calories and none of the fruit FIBRE.

The F-Plan diet has two special features: it recommends foods with high-fibre content and a half pint of skimmed MILK daily. The milk is to assure adequate dietary MIN-ERALS, especially CALCIUM, the ABSORPTION of which may be hindered by fibre.

The fibre meets two main needs. First, it satisfies psychological hunger by increasing chewing and thus slowing down eating, and by increasing the bulk of food passing through the mouth and filling the stomach. Second, increased bulk also causes food to move through the intestines more rapidly reducing the risk of diseases of the gut such as CANCER of the colon and DIVERTICULITIS.

The average British diet contains about 20g of fibre a day. The F-Plan diet recommends a minimum of 35g and a maximum of 50g (see also DIET, BALANCED).

To help build up fibre intake, the diet includes a daily quota of 'Fibre-Filler', a muesli-like CEREAL consisting of BRAN in various forms, almonds and dried fruits sufficient to assure 15g of fibre a day. Other fibre-rich foods recommended include SOYA flour BREAD, tinned baked beans, peas and other PULSES and wholewheat pasta.

The diet requires both calorie and fibre counting. That is, the dieter is advised to eat between 1000 and 1500 Calories and between 35 and 50g of fibre each day. For those whose dieting is helped by measuring and counting, the F-Plan would seem to be particularly well-suited. There can also be little doubt that fibre produces bulk, and bulk helps to create a psychological sense of fullness. On the negative side, damage to the stomach lining or even in the intestines by very rough cereals such as whole bran does occur. Anyone with a history of stomach or duodenal ULCERS should consult a doctor before trying a fibre-based diet. Indeed, *The F-Plan* clearly warns all readers to check with a doctor 'before embarking on a dieting programme'.

FRUCTOSE DIET See BEVERLY HILLS DIET

FRUIT
1. The edible stalk, bud, flower or seed of plants. Thus, tomatoes, globe artichokes, asparagus and NUTS are all fruit from the botanical standpoint. Even in common usage, the word encompasses plant products as different as limes, strawberries, blackcurrants and pineapples, so an acceptable popular definition might be 2. the sweet-tasting parts of plants.

Using the second definition, fresh fruits are the dieter's friend. They are 80 to 90 per cent WATER and range in CALORIE content from a low in rhubarb to a high in bananas. Even bananas have only about 100 Calories per 125g (4oz). No fruits contain much FAT, and they are good sources of some MINERALS and VITAMIN C. Excepting apples, grapes, grapefruit, pears, strawberries and white melons, fruit is also a good source of vitamin A, and bananas, grapefruit and oranges also contain folic acid.

Dried fruit is much more calorific than fresh fruits because it contains much less water and proportionately more SUGAR. For example, 100g (3½oz) of fresh apricots has 28 Calories. The same weight of dried apricots provides 182 Calories. On the other hand, dried fruit is a better source of FIBRE: fresh apricots contain 2.1g of fibre per 100g of fruit compared to 24g per 100g of the dried fruit.

In the process of ripening, fruit changes COLOUR. STARCH and CELLULOSE are broken down to become sugar, usually fructose (fruit sugar) or glucose. Apples, pears and some other fruit also contain sucrose. The enlargement during ripening is partly due to water retention.

Most people like fruit because it is lightly flavoured and refreshing. All fruits contain weak ACIDS: ascorbic acid or vitamin C, citric acid in pineapple, raspberries, strawberries and the citrus fruits (oranges, lemons, limes and grapefruit), oxalic acid in rhubarb and strawberries (poisonous amounts of oxalic acid are contained in rhubarb leaves), malic acid in apples and plums and benzoic acid in cranberries. Fruit acids do not normally increase stomach acidity, but the taste may be too sharp for people with chronic digestive disorders.

The most important fruit vitamin is, of course, vitamin C, but the amounts vary greatly. Apples have from 2 to 30mg per 100g whereas oranges have between 35 and 80mg. Apple juice itself is not a good source unless the vitamin has been added in PROCESSING. During stewing or boiling, most of the vitamin C leaches into the water. It remains there, but prolonged cooking or storage can destroy it. Blanching fruit before freezing reduces storage losses. Some 60 per cent of vitamin C disappears in the process of bottling or canning. However, bottled or canned citrus fruit juices retain up to 90 per cent until the containers are opened. Then vitamin C vanishes in the air. Over half will be lost from an open can of orange juice in a week. 'Whole fruit' drinks, squashes and cordials contain almost no vitamin C unless it has been added.

Apples and pears when tinned may have added ANTIOXI-DANTS to prevent browning. PRESERVATIVES are permitted in bananas and citrus fruits to control mould growth.

Apples, apricots, bananas, pears and tomatoes are picked commercially before they ripen, and the ripening process is controlled by temperature, humidity and the use of ethylene gas, an analogue of a natural ripening HORMONE.

G

GALL BLADDER DIET

A low-fat diet (see PRITIKIN, SCARSDALE) designed to control the symptoms of gall bladder disease.

The gall bladder is a small sack just below the liver and attached to it. It stores and concentrates BILE. Passage of food from the stomach to the small intestine causes release of a HORMONE, cholecystokinin, which stimulates the gall bladder to contract, ejecting bile into the intestine.

Gall bladder disease is commonly caused by one of two related disorders: gall stones and inflammation. Gall stones are insoluble deposits often of CHOLESTEROL precipitated out of the bile. The cause of this malfunction is seldom clear. Inflammation may be caused by the stones or by an infection. The symptoms of both disorders include pain and indigestion, jaundice and an intolerance for fatty food.

Gall bladder diets may control the symptoms. They cannot correct the underlying disorder, nor will diet alone improve jaundice.

GARLIC

(*Allium sativum*) One of the most widely-used cooking HERBS popularly believed to have both curative and prophy-lactic properties. Garlic is rich in CARBOHYDRATES containing about 130 Calories per 100g (3½oz).

Egyptian records from 5500 B.C. and Sanskrit, Roman and Hebrew literature refer to garlic. It is said to be an antibacterial drug like an antibiotic, to lower high blood pressure by dilating blood vessels and to improve the balance between useful and harmful bacteria in the intestines; and to distract werewolves.

A broad-leaved variety of the same species grows in Britain, but the root is a single, fleshy tuber like a horse-radish rather than the familiar clump of cloves.

GELATINE

A PROTEIN obtained by boiling bones or connective tissue. When it cools, the gelatine sets.

Gelatine is the basis of all sweet jellies. Those made commercially contain CARBOHYDRATE, COLOUR and FLAVOUR but no FRUIT juice and therefore no VITAMINS. Gelatine itself lacks the essential AMINO ACID tryptophan, and contains very little PHENYLALANINE. Thus, it has limited nutritive value.

GINSENG

(*Panax ginseng*) Originally, a Chinese HERB. An American ginseng comes from a related species, *Panax quinquefolium*. After being soaked and dried, the root is eaten. Alternatively, it may be boiled to make an infusion like TEA.

Manchurian ginseng was at one time considered to be so

superior to all others that it became scarce. The Chinese emperor, it is said, forbade its collection.

Ginseng is reputed to cure impotence and frigidity. It is also supposed to add to one's general sense of well-being. Psychic benefits such as these may well accrue to a user who is already convinced that the root will help him or her. There is no hard evidence, however, that ginseng can cure or prevent any conditions or diseases.

GLUCODIN ®

A SUGAR substitute and SLIMMING AID. It has 340 CALORIES per 100g (3½oz) or about 20 per cent less than sugar. It is also much less sweet than sugar so that more may be used. Glucodin is made from dextrose, another kind of sugar, to which VITAMIN C is added.

GLUTEN

A PROTEIN which stretches when mixed with WATER and kneaded; therefore, useful for bread- and cake-making. Gluten is present in wheat and rye and to a lesser extent, in oats and barley.

When flour is stored, gluten toughens and becomes more elastic. The process can be hastened by improvers added to the flour, a process used in commercial bread-making (see BREAD).

People who are sensitive to gluten may develop COELIAC DISEASE. The best treatment is a gluten-free diet. Gluten protein can be replaced by the protein in EGGS and MILK.

GLYCOGEN

A complex CARBOHYDRATE, the natural storage form in animals of the SUGAR, glucose. Also called animal STARCH because starch is the analogous storage form in plants. However, glycogen is also found in rice and some other plants.

During the DIGESTIVE PROCESS or in the liver, all carbohydrates are converted to glucose. That which is not used immediately for ENERGY is linked together by the action of ENZYMES into long chains of glycogen. Whether glucose is left free to circulate in the blood for immediate use or taken up for storage depends on interactions among several HORMONES. Three are of particular importance, and two of these are pancreatic hormones: glucagon promotes storage and insulin facilitates the uptake of glucose by cells thus calling for more to be made available in the blood. The third is adrenalin (US: epinephrine) which also promotes the breakdown of glycogen. The whole story of glucose control remains to be worked out, but its importance to the body's economy is underlined by the complexity of its regulation.

Adult bodies contain about two pounds of glycogen. Muscle cells have their own reserves. In the normal sedentary living pattern, however, glycogen in the liver is broken down to provide energy between meals.

GOUT

A disease principally of the joints with arthritis-like symptoms including stiffness, swelling and pain. Traditionally, gout has been associated with diet. Although food and drink may play a role in the development of the disease, other causes are important though poorly understood. However, most gout patients are overweight.

There is a familial tendency toward gout, and it is more common in men than women. Both facts imply a genetic predisposition to the disorder.

The pain and swelling are caused by deposits of crystals formed from uric acid, a common waste product in our bodies. Uric acid is carried by the blood and secreted through the kidneys in the urine. At normal blood levels (about 0.02 per cent), uric acid is a liquid, but in some people, the quantity of uric acid in the blood rises. It then precipitates in the form of crystals. In Britain, about three in every 100 people have abnormally high levels of uric acid in their blood, but only about three in every 1000 have gout, a discrepancy that underlines the problem of determining what causes the disease.

Uric acid crystals may also damage the kidneys and arteries. Indeed, these are the most serious complications of chronic gout. The more familiar symptoms are not directly caused by the crystals, but the crystals deposited in joints cause immune defence cells (see ALLERGY) called phagocytes to collect near them. Phagocytes are part of the body's natural machinery for removing the crystals, but they damage cells in the joints. Because of the damage, they release inflammatory chemicals which produce the symptoms.

Uric acid is the breakdown product of substances called purines. Not only do purines occur in every body cell, for example as part of the genetic material DNA, but they are a constituent of most food. Many FISH AND SHELLFISH, fish roe, MEAT extracts, offal, YEAST and yeast extracts are especially rich sources of purines. ALCOHOL contains no purines, but in the blood it interferes with excretion of uric acid. This is no doubt what underlies the old belief that gout is caused by high living. In all events, people with gout and families in which gout occurs are probably well advised to regulate their intake of purine-rich food and of alcohol.

Incidentally, CAFFEINE is a purine, but fortunately for COFFEE and TEA drinkers, the body cannot convert it to uric acid. Therefore, neither beverage is proscribed for gout sufferers.

Anyone with gout will benefit from dietary restriction. For example, the less weight the patient carries, the less strain on foot and leg joints, the most common sites of gouty attacks. What is more, the attacks themselves may be less frequent if the patient loses weight. However, today the symptoms are commonly controlled by drugs which allow more dietary freedom.

H

HEALTH FOOD

1. Any food or drink containing NUTRIENTS and free of dangerous poisons. 2. Any food sold in a health food shop.

Note that WATER, containing neither nutrients nor

poisons, is essential to health, a truism which gives a desirable perspective to the emotive phrase, 'health food'. Thus, under the narrowest definition (2, above), rhubarb is a health food providing it has been grown 'organically'; that is, without artificial fertilizers or pesticides. Yet rhubarb contains oxalic acid, a substance which occurs in such quantity in the leaves of rhubarb plants that they make you very sick indeed. In the edible stalk, the poison concentration is not dangerous but, in theory, eating too much rhubarb could poison you.

Another example of the hidden dangers in a popular phrase: health foods are often described as WHOLEFOODS, unprocessed, nothing added and nothing removed. Raw MILK is a whole food. The process of pasteurization removes from milk certain common but infectious germs. TAPIOCA contains cyanide which is removed by processing the cassava root from which the food comes. We do well not to be carried away by a phrase.

Health foods (definition 2) tend to be more expensive than ordinary foods and not simply because the shops that sell them charge what the trendy traffic will bear. Farming without pesticides and using only organic manure, horse manure or night soil as in China, for example, means lower yields per acre. Despite the disastrous effects of DDT, no one has yet shown that the new generation of pesticides, to say nothing of synthetic manure, damages either the environment or the consumer's health (see also POISON, FOOD). Given a choice, most of the people in this underfed world would be eager to risk it anyway in return for another spoonful of rice. The very cost of health foods implies a disregard for the needs of the great majority of our fellows.

Health food movements have contributed to popular awareness of good nutrition and a balanced DIET, however. For example, the BRAN and roughage freaks realized the value of FIBRE long before the professionals acknowledged it, even though some of the early apostles went overboard (a bowl-full of sand could be found on some sideboards on the theory that a spoonful a day kept you regular!). The health food movements have also taught the importance of fresh as opposed to processed foods, pointing out that ADDITIVES may reach unacceptable levels if you eat nothing but packaged puddings and MEAT pies. They showed that fresh food is usually cheaper in season and emphasized what we should all know: properly prepared fresh food usually tastes better. On the debit side are the HONEY addicts and the VITAMIN E faddists, but all extreme claims are suspect in politics, love and food. You can drown in too much water.

HERB

Mainly the leaves of a plant containing aromatic OILS, but also the stamens (as in saffron), roots (HORSERADISH), seeds (pepper, cardamom, poppy) and fruit (vanilla, cinnamon) of a plant. But are the latter not spices? Neither usage nor the *Oxford English Dictionary* give clear guidance. For example, kelp, the leaves of a seaweed, is a common Chinese spice. Garlic is a root or corm. Though it is usually thought of as an herb, mustard (herb or spice?) is a seed. One authority suggests that herbs originate in Europe and spices in the Far East with some overlap in the Middle East (R. J. Taylor, *Food Additives*, 1980). Pronunciation of the word 'herb' is also open to question. The British tend to use the 'h' whereas Americans often omit it. One can say with certainty only that both herbs and spices add FLAVOUR to food.

The nutritive value of herbs is similar to that of other green VEGETABLES with one important difference: we eat very small quantities of herbs so their nutritional contribution is minute. Only watercress and parsley are used in sufficient quantities to contribute to the diet, and they are both valuable supplements. Two tablespoons, about 2g, of chopped parsley contains a tenth of the recommended adult daily intake of VITAMINS A and C, though much of the vitamin C is lost in the chopping process. Dried herbs contain almost no vitamins, but other nutrients remain.

HERBALISM

The art of using HERBS as medicines. Herbalist practices have an ancient and honourable history in Britain, the

Middle East, India, China and north America. In fact, no civilization has lacked a herb-based medicine. Many herbs unquestionably display palliative value, and a few may cure some conditions. In this respect, herbs are not unlike modern drugs, natural and synthetic. Many control symptoms, and a few like the antibiotics actually cure. The difference is that the effects of modern drugs are more predictable than those of herbs. A measured dose can usually be related precisely to an effect, a relationship that rarely if ever exists in herbalism.

For the nutritive value of herbs, see HERB.

HONEY
The nectar of flowers collected by bees and concentrated by the loss of WATER and chemical changes.

Honey is probably the oldest SWEETENER. Sweeter than ordinary white SUGAR, sucrose, on a weight for weight basis, honey also has fewer CALORIES because 15 per cent of its weight is water. It also contains small amounts of PHOSPHORUS and POTASSIUM and traces of other MINERALS and VITAMINS B_2 and B_3. Claims that honey improves health or combats disease, however, are entirely without foundation.

Honeys vary in aroma because of the different flowers from which they are made. Indeed, a honey made from a rhododendron (*Azalea pontica*) that grows near Trabzon on the Black Sea coast of Turkey contain toxins that cause headache, vomiting and disorientation. It is believed to have poisoned Xenophon's soldiers, a catastrophe described in his *Retreat of the Ten Thousand*.

When they collect nectar, bees use an ENZYME, invertase, which converts the sucrose to dextrose and fructose. In the comb, the nectar loses water. Of course, it is stored by the bees as food for their larvae.

HORMONE
A chemical released by one group of body cells to change the behaviour of cells elsewhere in the body. Although there are some forty identified hormones, this entry will

describe only those connected with the DIGESTIVE PROCESS and food ABSORPTION.

Two hormones, cholecystokinin and gastrin, are directly involved in the digestive process. Cholecystokinin is synthesized by cells in the small intestine. They begin to produce the hormone when FAT enters the small intestine from the stomach. Cholecystokinin enters the blood and causes the gall bladder (see GALL BLADDER DIET) to discharge BILE.

Gastrin is secreted by cells in the stomach wall near the exit to the small intestine. Food and possibly also the sight or smell of food triggers secretion of gastrin. In parallel with nervous control from the brain, the hormone regulates synthesis of hydrochloric acid and probably also of pepsin by other stomach-wall cells. A third stomach hormone, enterogastrone, acts locally in the presence of fat to slow the emptying of the stomach.

Four hormones are involved in the use or storage of glucose, the SUGAR which is broken down to provide most of our ENERGY. They are adrenaline, glucagon, hydrocortisone and insulin. Two more hormones, calcitonin and parathormone, participate in the control of CALCIUM utilization. As its name implies, growth hormone helps to regulate growth, a function that it shares with thyroxine, a hormone secreted by the THYROID.

The release of adrenaline, growth hormone, hydrocortisone and thyroxine is controlled principally by the brain. The other hormones respond to local stimuli such as fat in the intestine (see gastrin, above). This point is of interest because hormones can be looked upon as a form of body-wide control like the nerves, working more slowly than the nerves but over a longer period.

Thyroxine, the sex hormones (which are not directly relevant to the utilization of food) and some others are occasionally recommended as dieting aids. Their use for this purpose is both dangerous and ineffectual. Hormones are powerful substances which must never be used except under direct medical supervision.

HORSERADISH

An HERB used as a flavouring, especially with MEAT. It has few CALORIES (59 per 100g/3½oz), average FIBRE content (8.3g per 100g) and is rich in MINERALS, especially CALCIUM and PHOSPHORUS, and VITAMIN C.

Horseradish sauce made with VINEGAR or WATER is also low in Calories, but if MILK or cream is used to moisten the ground root, the ENERGY content rises accordingly.

HUMECTANT, HUMEFACTANT

An ADDITIVE designed to retain WATER in food. Thus, it has an effect opposite to that of an ANTICAKING AGENT. BREAD and cakes in particular dry out quickly. Humectants lengthen their shelf-life.

These additives are also permitted in frozen chicken and FISH to which water is added. The effect is to increase weight as well as to prevent shrinkage. EEC regulations stipulate a maximum water pick up of 7.4 per cent by weight during POULTRY freezing.

The most common humectants are glycerol, a product of animal FAT, sorbitol, found in apples, peas and some berries, mannitol which is obtained from brown seaweeds, and propylene glycol, a synthetic chemical. Polyphosphate solutions are used to increase water content in fish and poultry.

HYPNOSIS

A trance-like state which differs in important respects from both sleep and waking. During hypnosis, the subject is responsive to suggestions made by the hypnotist and unless instructed to remember, will forget the period of hypnosis and suggestion. However, suggestions repugnant to the subject will not be accepted. Nor is it possible to hypnotize an unwilling subject, popular legends to the contrary notwithstanding. In fact, one out of every five people cannot be hypnotized even if he or she is willing.

Hypnosis may play a role in losing weight for some people, but only if their excessive eating is in some measure an hysterical response. Though the word, hysteria, comes

from a Greek word meaning uterus because the condition
was thought to be an exclusively female neurosis, it occurs
in both sexes. In common speech, it means histrionic. In
medical language, hysteria reflects the conversion of anxiety
into symptoms of physical illness. In a case of hysteria
related to over-eating, the patient may be anxious about his
inability to find a woman who wants to marry him. That
anxiety may be complicated by his fear of marriage, a
conflict within his own emotional life. He over-eats to
confirm his unattractiveness to women and at the same
time, to guarantee the perpetuation of his single state.
OBESITY in such a person is called a 'secondary gain'
because, despite its disadvantages, it reinforces and per-
petuates the underlying conflict. Most hysterics appear to
be good subjects for hypnosis, a fact used therapeutically
by Joseph Breuer and Sigmund Freud.

The hypnotist may be able to break into the hysterical
circle by suggesting that the patient will now find cream
buns or SUGAR in TEA distasteful. Such specific suggestions
often work whereas generalized instructions to go on a diet
do not. There is a risk, however, which any reputable
doctor will have considered before undertaking hypnosis: if
over-eating provides a secondary gain, the patient may well
try to replace it with another behaviour pattern which is
even more unpleasant or dangerous to his health; for
example, ALLERGY-like reactions to soap which cause him
to stop washing. The risk that the patient may substitute
some new kind of disagreeable behaviour for over-eating
is the best argument against casual use of untrained
hypnotists.

Your GP should be able to judge whether hypnosis
could help you with your weight problem. If the GP
does not practise hypnotism, a doctor who does will be
recommended.

I

IODINE

An essential TRACE ELEMENT which must be obtained from food. Sea FISH, seaweed and iodized SALT are the only adequate sources.

Iodine is leached out of fish when it is boiled but can be recovered if the WATER is used to make a sauce. Frying, grilling and baking do not significantly reduce iodine. Seaweed is unusual food in the western diet, but it is much more common in the Far East. In Britain and America, iodized salt is the most common source of iodine. Iodized salt is ordinary sea salt to which a small amount of iodine has been added. About half the average daily salt intake will provide the recommended daily dose of iodine for a healthy, non-pregnant adult, 100 micrograms (a microgram is a millionth of a gram).

Iodine is needed to synthesize the THYROID HORMONES, thyroxine and tri-iodothyroxine. Each molecule of the former contains four iodine atoms whereas the latter contains only three, as its name suggests. The thyroid hormones regulate growth and METABOLISM. If a pregnant woman eats too little iodine, her infant may be mentally retarded, deaf and mute. In the absence of adequate iodine, the thyroid gland swells forming a goitre. Goitre used to be common in areas where soil content of iodine is low such as the Cotswolds, the Mendips and Derbyshire. Such disorders are now rare in the developed world thanks to the practice of iodizing salt.

IONAMIN ® See DUROMINE

IRON

An essential MINERAL easily obtained in adequate amounts from the standard British and American diet. There are two important exceptions, however: during pregnancy and after injuries causing significant loss of blood, iron supplements may be necessary.

The richest food sources of iron are cockles and mussels, winkles, liver, kidney, black sausage and Bovril. Corned beef, heart, hare and pheasant are only slightly less valuable followed by beef, duck, oysters, whelks and SOYA BEANS. By and large, FISH and MEAT are better sources than VEGETABLES even though many fresh vegetables contain almost as much iron as beef. Part of the mineral is leached out during boiling though it can be recovered if the water is used for soup; but the iron in vegetables is less readily absorbed than that in animal food (see ABSORPTION). For example, in wholewheat flour, phytic acid impairs iron as well as CALCIUM absorption. On the other hand, VITAMIN C enhances absorption. A glass of orange juice at breakfast increases the iron obtained from morning EGGS and toast. Fresh FRUIT, SUGAR and dairy products contain almost no iron, however.

The average western diet provides about 10mg of iron a day. Most of us absorb only about 1mg or 10 per cent of this, enough for adult men, but about half the daily requirement for women and growing children. Women must replace blood lost every month, and children are adding to the amount of blood in their bodies as they grow. If a woman is pregnant or breast feeding, her needs will be even higher. Fortunately, these additional needs may be met because, in these circumstances, the body absorbs much more of the iron contained in food, up to a third of the total. The physiological machinery behind this topping-up operation is not understood.

The adult body normally contains between 3 and 4g of iron, about two-thirds of it in haemoglobin. Haemoglobin is the molecule inside red blood cells that carries oxygen and gives the cells their colour. The remaining iron is either involved in ENERGY production by cells or it is in transit in the blood. Very little body iron is lost except through haemorrhage or during menstruation, but a half teaspoonful of blood contains about 1mg of iron. So small a loss doubles the normal daily requirement. Most of the iron in haemoglobin is recirculated. In fact, the only normal loss in men occurs through the sloughing of skin or other surface cells.

Old people must be careful to ensure that their diets contain enough iron of the type that can be absorbed. Corned beef, sardines and pilchards are good sources, and they are also easy to prepare and chew.

The lack of adequate iron causes iron-deficiency anaemia. The patient has too few functioning red blood cells, and the body tissues receive too little oxygen. Tiredness, weakness and general malaise may be early symptoms. Later, the person takes on a bluish colour about the lips, has trouble breathing and can suffer a heart attack. Severe anaemia is extremely dangerous and must be corrected, if necessary by iron injections and blood transfusions. Other forms of anaemia are associated with VITAMIN deficiencies and with certain CANCERS. Iron poisoning from eating too much is rare. A few people inherit a condition in which they absorb too much iron which may be treated by blood letting. Alcoholics can accumulate excessive iron from cheap wine, a rich source. But the only real danger is to children who may be attracted to a bottle of pretty red iron pills; a few will do no harm but fifty could kill a child. Fortunately, there is a drug, desferroxamine, that acts as an antidote to iron poisoning whatever its cause.

IRRITABLE BOWEL SYNDROME
A disorder characterized by abdominal pain and diarrhoea without a demonstrable physical cause. The word 'syndrome' indicates that these signs and symptoms occur together and without other symptoms, for example, headache or fever.

Many authorities believe that irritable bowel syndrome is a hypersensitivity reaction due to a food ALLERGY. Carefully controlled scientific tests suggest that this may be true for a small minority of patients, three out of nineteen in one study. Psychological factors seem to be more prominent in most patients; that is, their symptoms are related to worry, depression or mild neurosis. In those few who have an allergy, however, if the cause can be identified, patients get better on diets free of the offending food.

J

JOULE (J)

A unit of measurement for work or ENERGY. One CALORIE equals 4184 Joules. However, a Calorie is a unit of energy in the form of heat only, whereas a Joule measures all forms of energy; e.g., electrical, chemical, nuclear.

Thus, one horsepower per hour = 2.685 MJ
one British Thermal Unit (BTU) = 1.055 kJ
one kilowatt hour = 3.6 kJ
one gram of FAT contains about 37 kJ
one gram of CARBOHYDRATE contains about 16 kJ
one gram of PROTEIN contains about 17 kJ
one gram of ALCOHOL contains about 29 kJ
1000 Joules = 1 kiloJoule (kJ)
1,000,000 Joules = 1 megaJoule (MJ)

The Joule is an SI unit; that is, Système International d'Unités. One Joule is equal to the work done when a force of 1 newton moves an object a distance of 1 metre. A newton (N) is the force needed to give an object weighing 1kg an acceleration of 1 metre per second per second.

The Joule was named for a British scientist, James Prescott Joule (1818–89), and the newton for Sir Isaac Newton (1642–1727).

K

KETONE

A compound formed in the body from the breakdown of FAT and used to produce ENERGY. In starvation or a disease such as DIABETES, too many ketones are formed. They

cannot be converted to energy and the excess causes body
fluids to become too ACID. This condition, called ketosis,
can lead to coma and death.

Ketosis reflects a state in which cells are being starved of
the energy-producing SUGAR, glucose. Fat and PROTEIN are
broken down to produce glucose. In the process, the
energy-producing machinery is subverted so that ketones
are formed which cannot be used up. Like sugar, ketones
are CARBOHYDRATES. Those formed by the body are aceto-
acetic acid, beta-hydroxybutyric acid and acetone. It has
been suggested that the 'odour of sanctity' associated with
starvation self-imposed by medieval holy men was really
the smell of acetone on their breath.

KWASHIORKOR

A form of MALNUTRITION in children associated with a diet
poor in PROTEIN and probably also lacking some VITAMINS.
The causes of the disease are unclear and may vary from
place to place. The symptoms include skin sores, muscle
wasting, weakness, puffiness due to WATER accumulation
and thin, reddish hair. The word, kwashiorkor, contains a
west African stem word meaning red.

The disease is widespread in tropical Africa, especially
among toddlers. After weaning, their staple diet is often
cassava (see CEREAL, TAPIOCA) which contains little protein.
Dried MILK products or other protein-rich food such as
SOYA can usually correct the symptoms of kwashiorkor but,
if the disease has gone too far, the child's digestive organs
may have degenerated to a point where ABSORPTION is
permanently impaired. These children will always remain
underdeveloped.

L

LABELLING

Two kinds of labelling of food products are regulated by
law or by a Code of Practice used as a guide by the Courts:

1. listing of ingredients; 2. claims about NUTRIENTS in the product or its value as a medicine or for slimming.

Almost all processed food must carry a list of ingredients. The exceptions are complete meals, BREAD, butter, CHEESE, flour and SUGAR confectionery including sweets and chocolates, fresh FRUITS and VEGETABLES and ice-cream. These foods are controlled by regulations specifying their composition. Very small containers are also exempt from the listing regulations. For example, an Oxo cube does not carry its contents, but the package of cubes does.

Ingredients are listed in decreasing order of weight, but again there are exceptions: mixed fruit and vegetables are listed alphabetically; WATER is not listed even if it is added; food like tinned fruit in syrup, VINEGAR or liquor may list the food first even though the liquid weighs more.

Excepting some ENZYMES and FLAVOURS, and substances not controlled by permitted lists, all ADDITIVES must be listed on the product. They may appear either in the form of the chemical name, for example, sulphur dioxide, or under a class name, for example, 'permitted PRESERVATIVE'. Additives permitted by EEC regulations have been given E (European) numbers and may be listed by these numbers. For a list of E numbers and the substances they represent, see Appendix II. Amounts included in the product must be stated with two exceptions: if the quantity of ANTIOXIDANTS and PRESERVATIVES used is less than 5 per cent of the permitted amounts, no quantification is needed. The word 'flavour' must be prominently presented separately from the list of additives if the flavour of the product derives largely from an additive; e.g., orange-flavoured, chocolate-flavoured. Amounts must be stated per 100g or 100ml. The following claims are permitted:

That the product supplies 'Energy', but only if it is a 'significant' source.

That the product supplies 'Protein', but only if it contains at least 3g/100g, or less than the protein in one EGG.

That the product supplies minerals, but only if it contains CALCIUM, IRON and IODINE.

That the product contains VITAMINS, but only if it contains vitamin A, B_1, B_2, B_3, C or D.

Added nutrients may not be listed on the label, however, unless the product contains enough of that nutrient so that one day's intake of the product provides a sixth of the recommended adult daily intake of that nutrient. The words 'rich' or 'excellent source of' may not be used unless the product contains half of the recommended daily adult intake.

Claims that a product can prevent or cure a disease are forbidden unless it contains all of the recommended daily intake of a nutrient directly related to that disease; for example, vitamin B_1 can prevent pellagra and is, therefore, related to it. Claims that a product has slimming properties are forbidden. A product may be labelled as part of a weight-reduction diet low in CALORIES, but the claim must be scientifically substantiated and the energy content of the ingredients separately listed. Many food products, especially those sold as part of a weight-reduction diet, are wholly synthetic. Even their nutrients may be manufactured rather than obtained from organic matter. Labelling does not indicate the ultimate source of the contents of a product. Phrases like 'country fresh' are mere advertising copy.

LACTATION
The process of MILK formation.

Human lactation is in every essential the same as cow lactation, or goat or sheep, though the nutrient content of milk differs from species to species. It is also noteworthy that, apart from size, before pregnancy there are no significant structural differences between the human female and male breasts. During pregnancy, lactation machinery in the form of specialized cells develop in the mother's breasts.

Failure of the human milk supply can be due to poor diet, but it is more commonly caused by emotional factors. Sometimes the milk dries up because a cracked, sore nipple destroys the pleasure of suckling. Whether or not a mother suckles her offspring depends very much on her attitude towards the feeding process. In other words, it is social and environmental rather than physiological factors which govern the mother's milk supply in most instances.

LECITHIN

1. A natural chemical compound in the body which acts as an EMULSIFIER in the blood and is found in other tissues, especially the white, protective covering of many nerves.
2. A common commercial emulsifier made from SOYA BEANS, peanuts or partially synthesized in the laboratory.

Natural lecithin is found in most foods. EGG yolk is the richest source containing about 10 per cent by weight. However, the body synthesizes all the lecithin it needs out of an AMINO ACID, methionine, SUGAR and FAT. Eating additional lecithin may mean eating too much fat and, therefore, too many CALORIES.

There is no evidence that lecithin promotes healthy nerves or protects against heart disease. On the other hand, if the body contained no lecithin, nerve and heart disorders would be the immediate consequence. Like CHOLESTEROL, lecithin is too important to the body's economy for its supply to be left to the whims of dietary fashion.

Lecithin is a phosphatide or phospholipid consisting of glycerol, fatty acids (see LIPID) and a small acidic molecule containing PHOSPHORUS.

LIMMITS ®

A SLIMMING AID, but a food, not a drug. Two Limmits biscuits are recommended by the manufacturer for a full meal containing 500 CALORIES (see VERY LOW CALORIE DIET).

Limmits consist of flour, SUGAR, FAT and small quantities of several other ingredients. In addition to CARBOHYDRATE, fat and PROTEIN, the biscuits contain CALCIUM, IRON and VITAMINS A, B_1, B_2, B_3, C and D.

LIPID

1. A FAT. The word 'fat' is commonly used in discussions of food and NUTRIENTS. 'Lipid' is used when the biochemistry of fats is under consideration. Thus, it is appropriate to

talk about the fat content of MILK rather than its lipid content. Conversely, CHOLESTEROL is usually classified as a lipid and not as a fat. Obviously, usages are customary rather than rigid, and some differences in usage may occur. For a precise definition, therefore, it is appropriate to add to this entry the chemical description of a lipid: 2. an organic substance insoluble in WATER but soluble in ALCOHOL, ether, chloroform or other fat solvents.

From the nutritional standpoint, lipid biochemistry is important for two reasons: 1. because lipids play three vital and quite distinctive roles in the body as sources of ENERGY, precursors of other vital chemicals and structural elements, and 2. because they also function as EMULSIFIERS in food PROCESSING. The molecular structure of lipids is relevant to these functions.

Like CARBOHYDRATES but not PROTEINS, lipids are small, simple molecules. They consist of a backbone which is an alcohol, glycerol, to which are attached one, two or three fatty ACIDS. In the body, lipids usually contain three fatty acids, and the molecule is called a triglyceride. Mono- (one fatty acid) and diglycerides are intermediate stages in the build up or breakdown of triglycerides.

The fatty acids all consist of carbon, hydrogen and oxygen arranged in carbon-hydrogen groups. The oxygen atoms appear only in the acidic carbon-hydrogen groups. These groups may be so organized that they are each connected by only one bond or chemical link, or they can be arranged so that two or more of the groups are connected by two bonds. More than two bonds between the groups in fatty acids is unusual. If the whole molecule is linked by single bonds, the fatty acid is saturated. If two bonds link any two groups, the fatty acid is unsaturated. The word unsaturated implies that the molecule is less stable or more reactive than saturated fatty acids in the sense that it 'strives' to become saturated. Saturated fatty acids are formed by animal including human tissues. The unsaturated fatty acids are formed almost entirely by plants. Neither humans nor other mammals can synthesize unsaturated fatty acids, but by and large, the saturated fatty acids provide the ingredients needed to make vital lipid derivatives such as cholesterol, HORMONES and LECITHIN. The one exception is an unsaturated fatty acid, linoleic acid, small amounts of which are essential and must be obtained from plant food.

Having thus briefly described the structure of lipid molecules, we can return to their functions. In the body, lipids are 1. sources of energy, 2. precursors of cholesterol, certain hormones (notably the sex hormones), lecithin and LOW-DENSITY LIPOPROTEINS, and 3. structural and protective. Their energy function has been discussed in detail in that entry and in the entry on FAT. Not only are the lipids essential precursors, but molecules such as cholesterol made from them are themselves vital parts of the body's chemical economy. In other words, although too much fat is not good for you (see DIET, BALANCED), you cannot do without it.

Lipids consisting of saturated fatty acids from animal products are associated with heart and circulatory disease, DIABETES and GOUT more frequently than lipids consisting of unsaturated fatty acids from plants. Despite pictorial expressions like furring of the arteries, no one knows why the connection exists or what exactly the saturated fatty acids do to help bring on the diseases. Because the immediate alleged culprits, cholesterol and low-density lipoproteins, are synthesized in our bodies and need not be obtained from food, it is now thought that the source of the trouble may be the blood-content of these lipids rather than dietary lipids as such. Lipids are also stored by cells where they are called upon to perform any of the functions noted above. Only if there is a rise in the blood-content of lipids, or of certain lipids, can damage to the blood vessels occur. It is possible that a similar relationship exists with metabolic disturbances such as diabetes and gout, but the regulator mechanism which should keep blood lipids within normal ranges is simply not understood.

In their structural and protective roles, lipid molecules perform perhaps their most common functions. For example, every cell in the body has a membrane separating it from other cells. The membrane consists basically of lipids. To be precise, the cell membrane is two lines of lipid molecules organized so that the water-soluble glycerol backbone of one faces the water-based liquid inside and outside the cell. The fatty-acid chains which are not water-soluble turn away from the inner and outer fluids, giving the membrane both viscousness and flexibility.

Lipids also form the white sheaths of myelin that wrap and protect nerves. In fat storage cells, moreover, lipids cushion delicate tissues such as the milk-forming glands of the breast against knocks and pressure.

In food processing, lipids are used as emulsifiers to improve and maintain the mixing of OILS with water-based substances such as VINEGAR (see also BILE, EGG). This role is an adaptation of the cell-membrane function just described because a single layer of lipid molecules is organized so that the glycerol backbone faces the water causing the fatty-acid tails to turn inward towards each other. The structure thus forms a ball or micelle which can enclose another lipid molecule.

You can observe this molecular layering of lipids yourself. Gently pour a teaspoon of oil on the surface of water in a glass. The oil should spread out thinly and evenly across the surface of the water forming a film just one molecule thick. Now shake the glass or stir the contents. Tiny oil bubbles will form out of part of the film. They are micelles. At the same time, part of the remaining surface film may seem to thicken, possibly because it has now formed a membrane-like bilayer of lipid molecules.

Lipids are also relevant to food processing because the unsaturated fatty acids tend to become rancid, as they do in butter, for example. Chemically, the relatively unstable molecule takes up more oxygen and becomes more acidic. ANTIOXIDANTS are designed to delay rancidity.

LOW-CARBOHYDRATE DIET
Any diet that supplies ENERGY in the form of FAT or PROTEIN in place of CARBOHYDRATE. As slimming diets, low-carbohydrate regimens are no better than meals containing

about the same amount of energy from BREAD or potatoes, both primarily carbohydrate foods. On the other hand, processed carbohydrates in the forms of SUGAR, pastry and confectionery are among the most obvious causes of overweight. For some people, therefore, it makes sense to combine weight loss with low-carbohydrate intake.

As with any other kind of quick-cure diet, certain warnings apply to the low-carbohydrate variety. Excessive WATER loss should be avoided. The dieter will also have to find ways to overcome the constipation that often accompanies lower food intake, especially if by cutting out carbohydrates, he or she also reduces FIBRE consumption. Finally, it is always important to beware of the clever diet that isn't. Eliminating useful foods containing carbohydrate may simply lead to their replacement by others that are less useful.

Low-carbohydrate slimming may be fairly slow. The diets often involve eating vast amounts of FRUIT (see BEVERLY HILLS DIET). Fruit contains significantly more water on a weight-for-weight basis than most other foods. It avoids the risk from water loss but, on the other hand, water loss is often the first source of weight loss. If your diet stresses fruit to the virtual exclusion of other foods, your water intake actually rises at the same time that your CALORIE consumption falls. You will lose weight, but it may not seem like it at first.

When you cut out carbohydrates, moreover, your body will obtain its energy from fats and proteins in the food you are allowed. Some low-carbohydrate diets are more deceptive than others, though, because their authors recognize how psychologically important a sweet may be to many of us. In order to assure that a low-carbohydrate dieter will stick to the prescribed regimen, therefore, the author may throw the reader a sugary bone: you can have your chocolate bar or your pastry and lose weight too.

Of course, you can see through this stratagem. If you eat three meals in a day with a total of 1100 Calories, you can also eat a Mars bar containing another 400 Calories and end up with a weight-reducing diet. Thus, a low-carbo-hydrate diet can work and still leave room for the daily treat that may make it all seem more bearable to the dieter.

If you look at dieting in this way, you can see how easy it is either to reduce your Calorie intake by another 25 per cent (1100 from meals + 400 from the sweet = 1500) or to add 400 Calories to your meals in such interesting and useful foods as a piece of bread (about 80 C), ½oz butter (about 120 C) or 4oz ice-cream (about 200 C). All three of these foods contain some vitamins and minerals as well as proteins and fats, whereas the Mars bar offers you primarily sugar and fats.

LOW-DENSITY LIPOPROTEIN (LDL)

A form of FAT circulating in the blood which is associated with heart and circulatory disease. There is statistical evidence that patients with cardiovascular disease have relatively more LDLs than those who are normal. In the west, older people in particular tend to have higher LDLs than younger people. In places where heart and circulatory disease is less common, however, age is not associated with increased blood levels of LDLs suggesting that the causes of the diseases must include factors other than age.

Low-density lipoproteins are molecules made up of a LIPID combined with a PROTEIN and lower in density than other similar molecules, the latter being, *ipso facto*, high-density lipoproteins. Dietary lipids including CHOLESTEROL and LECITHIN tend to increase circulating LDLs, but the LDL molecules are synthesized in the body to facilitate the movement of lipids through the blood stream. Not being soluble in water-based fluids like blood, lipids would be less easily transported if they were not combined with proteins which are WATER soluble.

Synthesis of LDLs is a normal body function, more or less independent of the intake of dietary lipids. Problems may arise when they are not broken down quickly enough to keep the blood levels normal. There are at least four categories of LDLs circulating in the blood, moreover. In the UK, only one of these, Type IV low-density lipoprotein, is associated with cardiovascular disease. Clearly, despite the apparent connection, we are dealing with a factor that is poorly understood and which has only an indirect connection with what we eat. Nevertheless, it is perhaps wisest to decrease total fat intake and to substitute unsaturated fats for saturated fats whenever possible. See DIET, BALANCED, LIPID, OBESITY.

M

MACROBIOTIC

A complete dietary system built on the exclusive consumption of unprocessed, natural foods in suitable combinations. Foods may be cooked. Seasoning may be used only if it adds some NUTRIENT to the dish. Macrobiotic diet includes animal as well as vegetable products and should not be confused with VEGAN or VEGETARIAN diets.

The system is said to grow out of the Zen Buddhist interpretation of the world. Macrobiotics was originated by a Japanese, Georges Ohsawa (1893–1966), who urged commonsense application of the ancient, pre-Buddhist Chinese yin and yang principles to food choice. For example, in cold climates, warming yang foods such as FISH, EGGS, buckwheat, rice and VEGETABLES should be eaten. Conversely, in the tropics, the thinner, more feminine yin foods such as salads, oats, wheat, HONEY and FRUIT are advised. Note that some foods such as rice and raw vegetables can be either yin or yang depending on their combination with other foods, the calendar periods when they are eaten and other factors.

Macrobiotic diets are intended to vary with the local food traditions. Thus, Scots eat oats and herring whereas Bengalis eat rice and fish, and Eskimos MEAT and blubber. Modern transportation permits more varied diets, but processed foods are forbidden.

Whole grain CEREALS such as wheat, corn, oats and rye comprise the main elements in every macrobiotic diet, and SOYA BEANS are highly recommended. Sweets should be natural: for example, honey is acceptable but refined SUGAR is not. Only TEA made from locally-available roasted grains, beans or roots such as BURDOCK or DANDELION is permitted, though how this stricture affects tea in Sri Lanka or COFFEE in the Kenyan hills is not clear. In any case, the use of liquids is restricted, a rule which may easily fly in the face of medical advice to people whose disorders range from the common cold to amoebic dysentery. Treatments for both require large quantities of liquid. As with other dietary regimens, a doctor's opinion may be important before starting a macrobiotic diet, especially during pregnancy, but a macrobiotic diet is likely to be well-balanced nutritionally. It should also provide adequate FIBRE. However, it may be expensive.

MAGNESIUM
An essential MINERAL easily obtained in adequate amounts from the average western diet. Magnesium is needed in tiny quantities by ENZYMES involved in ENERGY storage, and it is also necessary for the proper functioning of muscle and nerves.

The best sources are wheat germ, BRAN and wholegrain CEREALS, though phytic acid (see BREAD) in cereals interferes with ABSORPTION of magnesium as it does with CALCIUM and IRON. SOYA BEANS, winkles, shrimps, whelks and instant COFFEE powder are also good sources for the mineral. The British recommended adult daily intake is 300mg (US: 450mg), but more is required during pregnancy and breast feeding.

Severe diarrhoea and MALABSORPTION caused by disorders such as COELIAC DISEASE can dangerously reduce magnesium stores in the body. The mineral is normally held in bone, but if the supply becomes exhausted, the result can be lethargy, depression and even a fatal heart attack.

MALABSORPTION
A failure of ABSORPTION caused by disease or a malfunction in the DIGESTIVE PROCESS. Malabsorption may affect one or more NUTRIENTS, or it can be general, affecting all nutrients

and WATER. General malabsorption is often seen in gastro-
enteritis and characterizes cholera. In such diseases, the
patient suffers from severe and persistent diarrhoea which
can become life-threatening.

Some kinds of malabsorption are probably genetic in
origin. They are the result of a missing or malfunctioning
digestive ENZYME. COELIAC DISEASE is an example of this
kind of disorder. Intolerance to CARBOHYDRATES may take
the form of an inability to absorb the MILK sugar, lactose, a
condition inherited by some people from India and Pakis-
tan. Similarly, some people lack a substance called intrinsic
factor which should be synthesized by cells in the stomach.
They cannot absorb VITAMIN B_{12}.

In the absence of BILE and in some other conditions,
FAT may not be absorbed. Vitamins A, D, E and K are
fat-soluble, and in these circumstances, they are poorly
absorbed. Fat malabsorption may lead to a fatty diarrhoea
which can cause loss of another vitamin, folic acid, and
MINERALS such as CALCIUM and IRON. A low-fat diet may
control the symptoms, but it may also be a low-energy
diet, hastening weight loss. The patient will need both
vitamin and mineral supplements.

There are far too many malabsorption disorders to list
them all here with useful information about their symptoms
and causes. Suffice it to say that if you note any unusual
change in your stool that persists, a doctor's advice should
be sought. This is especially true in the case of small
children and during pregnancy.

MALNUTRITION

Bad nutrition. A condition affecting anyone whose diet is
not balanced, whether because they have too little of one or
more NUTRIENTS, or as is more commonly the case in the
UK and the US, because people eat too much of one or
more nutrients. Among the minority of the world's population where affluence prevails, malnutrition is a condition
of over-eating. Among the majority of the world's peoples,
malnutrition remains a condition associated with poor diet
or even starvation. Malnutrition may also be caused by

disease, as in MALABSORPTION. Diseases of malnutrition can originate with either excess intake (for example, heart and circulatory disease) or with poor diet (for example, iron deficiency anaemia).

The most serious malnutritional diseases may once have been such disorders as scurvy and pellagra caused by VITAMIN deficiencies. Now that the importance of vitamins, MINERALS and other nutrients is understood, however, malnutrition reflects either poverty or stupidity. Poverty affects far more people: 500 million children suffer each year from PROTEIN malnutrition (see KWASHIORKOR). As a cause of malnutrition, however, stupidity will be much more familiar to the readers of this book, unfortunately. Very few of us do not know that a diet of hamburgers and chips is both expensive and damaging to the health. Naturally, the present reader and I are excepted, but too many of our neighbours go right on eating too many fats and too little FIBRE despite knowing better.

MALT EXTRACT

A sweet, viscous extract from germinated and dried barley, oats or wheat. The sweetness comes from a SUGAR, maltose, found in these CEREALS. The sugar gives malt extract high ENERGY value. It adds a pleasant FLAVOUR to malt bread, malted drinks and barley sugar as well as to BEER. Because it is easily absorbed, malt extract may be useful for feeding patients with tuberculosis or even infantile cholera.

MARASMUS

Starvation in young children. Typically, it occurs in the early months of life when the mother is no longer able to breast feed, and there is no adequate alternative food supply. The child becomes wizened with a swollen belly and no ENERGY. Death usually follows an infection that the child cannot withstand.

If food is supplied in time, there may be full recovery. Unfortunately, no one knows at what point even a balanced diet will fail to restore normal growth.

Marasmus should not be confused with KWASHIORKOR, a form of MALNUTRITION associated with shortages of PROTEIN and VITAMINS, though both diseases are endemic in central Africa and some other third-world countries.

MARGARINE

An emulsion (see EMULSIFIER) of FAT and WATER with added COLOUR, FLAVOURS and, usually, VITAMINS, developed as a butter substitute. Margarine may contain up to 10 per cent butter by weight.

It was invented by a French chemist, H. Mege-Mouries, in 1869 as a cheap spread. Today, it often costs about the same as butter. Because FISH OILS are among its constituents, margarine has more vitamin D than butter. It should be eaten instead of butter by older people, Asian immigrants to Britain and others who may need more vitamin D in their diets. Unless butter is added, moreover, margarine is usually free of CHOLESTEROL though its lipid content varies with the fats available at the time for its manufacture. Thus, animal oils contain cholesterol, for example, but VEGETABLE oils do not.

Polyunsaturated fats are believed to be more easily used and disposed of by the body than saturated fats (see LIPID). Hard margarines contain about the same quantities of both as butter (about 5 per cent unsaturated and 95 per cent saturated), but the softer the margarine, the more polyunsaturated fats it contains.

Margarine and butter also have the same CALORIE content. Spreads advertised as 'low-fat' have more water than the 16 per cent by weight permitted in margarine. Therefore, they contain about half the Calories in margarine or butter. Their vitamin A and D content is about the same. Vitamin E is often added to margarine and other spreads, though not of course to butter. At least 80 per cent of margarines must be fats, but under existing regulations, the fats included need not be listed. Margarines may also contain ANTIOXIDANTS, emulsifiers, skimmed MILK and SALT.

MAZINDOL See TERONAC

MEAT

The flesh of animals other than FISH and POULTRY, used as
food. Meat is not the oldest human food if we judge by
archaeological evidence from remains such as bones, but it
is also one of the most easily digested and best absorbed.
Though there may be economic and moral arguments
against meat eating, all healthy humans benefit from a
small amount of meat, perhaps no more than two ounces
each day.

Curiously, a great many taboos have been associated with
meat consumption in different times and places while there
have been very few connected with plants. Two major
religions, Islam and Judaism, forbid the eating of pork;
none forbids non-poisonous plant food. There are probably
two reasons: meat may become toxic and yet have no
obvious bad smell or taste. For example, the parasite
causing trichinosis, a fatal infestation, cannot be observed
in pork with the naked eye and can only be killed by long
cooking at high temperatures, a culinary feat not easily
performed with primitive cooking fires. In the second place,
there has always been a proscription against cannibalism,
though it did not necessarily extend to enemies of the tribe.
Thus, meat taboos have a rational history whether or not
they remain sound today.

The moral argument against meat consumption, however, differs from the ancient taboos. It holds that humans
have no right to kill other animals or, conversely, that
other animals have as much right as we do to live out their
lives in security except for competition from their own
kind. Comment on the moral argument is beyond the brief
of this *Dictionary*.

The economic argument against meat eating recognizes
that the biological process of converting plant to animal
flesh is inefficient: only about a tenth of the grain used as
feed, for example, is returned as meat. Yet disproportion-
ately large proportions of the world's CEREALS are diverted
to animal food, the product of which is expensive and

nutritionally unnecessary. The argument does not deny that meat is food to eat and good for you. It holds that meat production is economically dubious in the face of persistent world food shortages. Therefore, to conserve meat and the resources that go into its making, it should be mixed with cereals in traditional recipes such as pastas, dumplings and pies.

Meat is an excellent source of ENERGY, MINERALS, PROTEIN and B VITAMINS. FAT provides most of the energy. All meat has from 1 per cent to 3 per cent invisible fat, but visible fat can be as high as 60 per cent, for example, in streaky bacon. Lean meat contains less than 20 per cent fat. The CALORIE content of beef which is a third fat is roughly twice that in 100 per cent lean beef. Meat fats contain CHOLESTEROL and saturated fatty acids (see LIPID). Beef and lamb have a higher proportion of saturated to unsaturated fatty acids than pork.

Meat is a good source of three minerals, IRON, POTASSIUM and PHOSPHORUS. About a third of the iron is in a chemical state that permits it to be absorbed and used by the body. Red meat contains more iron than white meat such as veal, rabbit and pork. Liver, kidney and black sausage are particularly rich sources. If for no other reason than its iron content, pre-menopausal women should eat some meat because the blood they lose each month must be replaced.

Meat protein is of high quality because it contains all the essential AMINO ACIDS. During pregnancy and growth, it is especially useful. In male adults and non-pregnant women, however, protein not used to maintain tissue is converted to energy, a wasteful use of a relatively rare NUTRIENT. Liver and kidney are exceptional because they contain vitamin A, the only fat-soluble vitamin found in meat. They are also especially good sources of folic acid and B_{12}. Pork is richer in B_1, thiamin, than other meat.

Fresh and frozen meats may not contain ANTIOXIDANTS, added COLOUR or PRESERVATIVES excepting that in Scotland in summer, sulphur dioxide is permitted as a preservative in mince. It may also be used at any time of year throughout

Britain in sausages and other cereal-containing meat products that must be cooked.

TENDERIZERS are permitted providing they are listed on a label on the package or near unpackaged cuts. Vitamins C and B_3, niacin, preserve colour and may be used for this purpose in cured bacon and ham, but they too may not be added to fresh or frozen meat.

Meat may contain traces of antibiotics or hormones that were fed to the animal. Permissible levels of these drugs are now controlled throughout the EEC but not yet in the US. Regulation has become imperative for two reasons: antibiotics absorbed at random by meat eaters were increasing the probability that bacteria resistant to the drugs would emerge – an extremely serious medical problem. The hormones presented a different problem which can be exemplified by the case of diethylstilbesterol (DES). It is a compound related to the sex hormones which was used to encourage growth in cattle. Now, DES is associated with the appearance of breast cancer in the daughters of women who ate meat containing it. Experience with antibiotics and hormones together with the risk that POISONS can be passed on through the food chain has led to rigorous controls on all animal feeds.

Frozen meats retain nutrients well although with time there is some loss of vitamin B_1, thiamin. Note that the drip from thawed meat will contain this vitamin and should if possible be used to make gravies or soup.

In meat products other than fresh and frozen meats, ADDITIVES are permitted. The quantity of meat varies from product to product, moreover, and is fixed by law. The following list shows the minimum permitted meat content of each product as a percentage of total content.

Product	Minimum percentage meat content
Canned beefburgers*	80
Canned meat*	95[†]
Curried meat*	35
Curried meat and rice*	15
Faggots	35

Product	Minimum percentage meat content
Frankfurters	75
Luncheon meat*	80
Meat and gravy*	75
Meat balls	35
Meat, gravy, stuffing and onion*	40
Pâtés	70
Pies, meat only	25
Pies, meat and vegetable	12.5
Pie fillings	35
Potted meat	95
Potted meat in jelly	70
Rice with meat, and similar	None
Rissoles	35
Salami	75
Sausage, pork**	65
Sausages, other	50
Spreads	70
Spreads 'requiring grilling'	None

* Meat may contain a maximum of 40 per cent fat meat.
† Canned hams, gammon, pork shoulder may contain more than 5 per cent jelly.
** 80 per cent of meat must be pork.

Other ingredients must be listed. Among the most widely-used fillers or non-meat additives to sausages, for example, are bread, rusk and novel or TEXTURED VEGETABLE PROTEIN. A flavouring agent, MONOSODIUM GLUTAMATE, the preservative, NISIN, and SALT are common meat additives.

METABOLISM
1. The sum of all chemical changes that make up the life of an organism at any time. 2. The chemical conversion of food to body tissue, ENERGY and, ultimately, waste.

It is sometimes said that A is fat because his metabolism is 'slower' than B's who is thin. Indeed, there are differences in basal metabolic rate; that is, the minimum energy expended at rest to maintain vital functions such as respiration, circulation, digestion, elimination and body temperature. These differences are probably inherited. Except in some diseases, however, the relation between basal metabolism and weight is at best unclear.

Weight differences are usually traceable to two factors: the amount of energy you use, for example, in work or EXERCISE, and the amount of food you eat. Some families run to fat, it is true; nevertheless, body shapes are more likely to be related to energy expenditure and food consumption than to the genes. Parents, especially mothers who are usually responsible for feeding the family, tend to see the ideal body shape in terms of their own self-image. There is good evidence that fat parents encourage their children to eat more than thin parents do with theirs. If the parents are averse to exercise and work at relatively sedentary occupations, moreover, their children often follow analogous life patterns. That is, they get less exercise than children of parents whose work is physically more taxing. The argument that one has a family tendency to overweight is a convenient fiction, except in the occasional, physically unusual individual.

On the other hand, some people are larger than others; they are taller and have bigger bones. The reasons are both genetic and environmental, but those reasons are not necessarily relevant to healthful body weight. As weight charts show (see OBESITY), bigger people obviously weigh more than smaller people regardless of their ages, work and diets. Some women have larger hip bones than others. Some men have larger rib cages. They are going to weigh more. In healthy people, metabolism is always adjusted by a number of different mechanisms, not all of which are clearly understood, to the needs of your bone structure and your energy output. What you do with your metabolism in the way of feeding it properly depends on two things: what you know about a balanced diet and your common sense.

METHYLCELLULOSE See CELEVAC, CELLUCON, NILSTIM

MIGRAINE See ALLERGY, FOOD

MILK
The secretion of the mammary glands which provides the first food for the newborn. Not surprisingly, milk is a well-balanced food containing essential NUTRIENTS. This is not

to say that a milk diet is recommended for adults. Many adults are actually no longer able to digest milk properly. They lack adequate supplies of an ENZYME, lactase, which splits milk SUGAR, lactose, into glucose and maltose. These two sugars can be absorbed but lactose cannot. CHEESE has no lactose but contains most of the other nutrients in milk and is more easily digested.

Diets like the F-PLAN do include milk, but only if it is skimmed. Whole milk is a rich food, high in CALORIES. A half-pint of cow's milk contains 130 Calories, roughly the same as four slices of white bread. Human milk has an even higher Calorie content because it contains more CARBOHYDRATE and FAT than cow's milk.

Species differences characterize all of the nutrients in milk. The faster the young of the species mature, the more MINERALS and PROTEIN in the mother's milk. At 2g per half-pint, the protein content of human milk is less than half that of cow's milk, and the CALCIUM, PHOSPHORUS and POTASSIUM content of human milk is also lower. Of the milk consumed by humans anywhere in the world, reindeer milk is highest in protein.

Cow's milk is always diluted before it is given to infants. The greater amount of phosphorus in cow's milk impairs human ABSORPTION of calcium and MAGNESIUM, and inadequate uptake of these minerals can cause serious nervous disorders. Cow's milk has half the VITAMIN C and less vitamin A than human milk, and human milk has more B vitamins. In fact, the amount of both vitamin C and D in human milk depends on the mother's diet. As in other foods, temperature and light affect the vitamin content of milk. Vitamin C is lost during storage and delivery of cow's milk. Vitamin B_2, riboflavin, is reduced by half by ultraviolet light if milk in a bottle is exposed to bright sun for only two hours.

The processing of milk, which is now all but universal, reduces its nutrients. Pasteurization, carried out in the UK largely by raising the temperature to 72 degrees for fifteen seconds, causes a 20 per cent loss of vitamin C. Other losses are smaller. UHT (Ultra High Temperature) is a sterilization process in which milk is heated to 130 degrees C for three to five seconds. It has about the same effect on nutrients as pasteurization. Evaporated or condensed milk is produced by removing WATER. Sugar can be added. The process reduces most vitamins but especially B_2, B_{12} and C. The oldest storage technique is drying, dating back to the thirteenth century when it was said to have been invented by the Mongol followers of Genghis Khan. Nutrient loss is also about the same as it is in pasteurization.

Cream is milk fat. Most milk contains about 3 to 4 per cent fat, and the fat content of different varieties of cream is fixed by law:

Type of cream	Percentage of fat content
Clotted	55
Double	48
Whipping	35
Sterilized	23
Single	18

EMULSIFIERS and STABILIZERS are permitted in whipped and sterilized cream. Whipped cream may also contain added sugar, and the PRESERVATIVE NISIN may be added to clotted cream. No other ADDITIVES are permitted. Sour cream is made from single cream by a process similar to that used for making YOGHURT.

If whole milk is churned or otherwise agitated, the solids coagulate forming butter and leaving a liquid called buttermilk despite the fact that it lacks all butter fat. Butter contains about 80 per cent fat and 10 per cent water. The remainder consists of milk solids, air and SALT. Additives may be COLOUR (carotene, or the artificial colouring agent, annatto), salt and, in butter sold for manufacturing or catering, ANTIOXIDANTS.

MINERAL
A metallic substance; in this context, an element which is an essential NUTRIENT and must be supplied in food.

Minerals build bones, teeth and nails. Tiny amounts are required for certain ENZYMES, but the bulk of the IRON in our bodies is used to form the PROTEIN, haemoglobin, which carries oxygen in red blood cells. Minerals are also needed for the proper functioning of nerves and muscles.

Traces (see TRACE ELEMENT) of as many as eighteen minerals have been found in the healthy human body, but seven are relatively more common: CALCIUM, iron, MAGNESIUM, PHOSPHORUS, POTASSIUM, SODIUM and SULPHUR. Others include copper, zinc, vanadium, cobalt and lithium.

MONOSODIUM GLUTAMATE

A substance that looks like ordinary SALT and enhances FLAVOUR. The chemical was synthesized in 1867, but its usefulness for flavouring was described in 1908 by a Japanese chemist, K. Ikeda. Though it is added to western foods, monosodium glutamate is more frequently used in Chinese cookery.

Excessive amounts affect some people unpleasantly. They suffer hot flushes around the neck, headache and sweating, symptoms called the Chinese restaurant syndrome because they were first identified among customers of such emporia. The syndrome only appears after a 'dose'of between 2 and 12 grams of monosodium glutamate, a quantity that a careless cook can easily surpass.

Monosodium glutamate is the SODIUM salt of an AMINO ACID, glutamic acid, just as ordinary salt is the sodium salt of hydrochloric acid (which is not an amino acid, of course).

MUESLI

A breakfast CEREAL commonly containing oats and dried FRUIT. Muesli originated in Switzerland, probably during the 1920s. Its popularity is due to its relatively high FIBRE content, about 7.4g per 100g (3½oz) (less than BRAN and some other cereals), combined with the tastes and textures of fruits and NUTS. It is customary to add MILK, but SUGAR should not be needed. The fruit contains natural sugar, and some commercial brands have added sugar already.

The list of contents on the package will show whether there is extra sugar in the muesli you are thinking of buying.

N

NETTLE
(*Urtica dioca*) Familiar as stinging nettle, but in May and June the new leaves can be lightly boiled (about ten minutes in half an inch of WATER), to produce a delicious, spinach-like VEGETABLE rich in MINERALS and VITAMIN C. The plant also contains B vitamins which are leached out in boiling but can be recovered if the water is used as stock for soup or sauces. Nettle may also be fermented to make a kind of BEER.

Claims abound for the nettle as a poultice, hair tonic and corrective for bowel troubles.

NILSTIM ®
A SLIMMING AID and laxative. It contains the same chemical, methylcellulose, as CELEVAC and CELLUCON, with the same effects. Nilstim is manufactured by a different company.

NISIN
A PRESERVATIVE interesting because it is a natural antibiotic found in some CHEESE. It is now used as a preservative for cheese, MEAT products, cream (see MILK) and canned foods subject to certain types of bacterial spoilage.

NITROSAMINE
A nitrogen-containing compound found naturally in many foods, both MEAT and VEGETABLES, and in our bodies. There is statistical evidence that nitrosamines may cause CANCER, possibly because they thwart the immune defences which should help to protect us (see ALLERGY, FOOD).

Since natural amounts of nitrosamines in food are very low, they are believed to be safe unless too much builds up in the body. However, the PRESERVATIVES, sodium nitrate and sodium nitrite, used to prevent contamination by the dangerous bacterium, *Clostridium botulinum*, may be converted to nitrosamines by our bodies. Therefore, there is a danger that the use of these ADDITIVES could raise the level of nitrosamines in food unacceptably. Nitrate-containing WATER may be an even greater risk.

NUTRIENT

A chemical constituent of food which can be utilized or stored for later use by body cells. A nutrient must be digested (see DIGESTIVE PROCESS) and absorbed (see ABSORPTION) before it can be used. It may provide ENERGY, possibly in the form of heat to maintain body temperature, structural components as in bone or muscle cells or functional components such as ENZYMES.

The major nutrient classes are CARBOHYDRATES including STARCH and SUGAR, FATS formed from fatty acids and made up of other LIPIDS such as CHOLESTEROL and PROTEIN which consists of some twenty AMINO ACIDS. In addition, a range of MINERALS, TRACE ELEMENTS and VITAMINS must be supplied in food. Minerals, the trace elements, vitamins, the fatty acid, linoleic acid, and eight of the amino acids are essential nutrients in that they cannot be synthesized in adequate amounts to meet body needs, if at all. The body can make all of the other nutrient sugars and starches, lipids and amino acids providing adequate carbohydrate, fat and protein and the essential nutrients are available in food.

Though it provides energy, ALCOHOL is usually considered to be a drug rather than a food. WATER and oxygen are actually essential for life, but they are not usually classed as nutrients.

NUTS

The seeds of trees and some other plants. Peanuts (ground nuts) are more closely related to beans and other PULSES.

All nuts are good sources of FAT, FIBRE, POTASSIUM, PROTEIN and the B VITAMINS with the exception of B_{12}. Chestnuts contain relatively more CARBOHYDRATE and less fat and protein. The energy content of nuts is high, ranging from 619 CALORIES per 100g (3½oz) in Brazil nuts to 351 C in the same amount of fresh coconut. The fat in coconut and cashew nuts is proportionately lower in polyunsaturated fats (see LIPID), and these nuts are the least satisfactory if you are looking for a low-cholesterol diet. In addition to potassium, nuts tend to be rich sources of CALCIUM, IRON and MAGNESIUM, but because they also contain phytic acid (see BREAD), these MINERALS are poorly absorbed. In sesame seeds, oxalic acid, the potential POISON found in spinach and rhubarb may also impair mineral ABSORPTION. Nuts are low in SALT unless they are salted during roasting.

Although they are often recommended as alternative sources of protein, nuts contain very little of the essential AMINO ACID, lysine. Almonds and peanuts are also poor sources of another essential amino acid, methionine. It is sensible, therefore, to supplement nuts with small quantities of MEAT protein.

With the exception of green walnuts, nuts lack vitamin C, and with the exceptions of pine kernels, pistachios and sesame seeds, vitamin A. Fictional accounts of lost explorers to the contrary notwithstanding, it is impossible to live indefinitely on a nut diet. Note also that nuts must be ground or well chewed if they are to yield up the NUTRIENTS they do contain. Otherwise, they pass through the digestive tract undigested, adding bulk but little else.

O

OBESITY

A disease characterized by an excess of body FAT. About 6 per cent of men and 8 per cent of women in the UK are classified as obese. According to a report published in *The Lancet* (1 October 1983, p. 784): 'There is increasing evidence that small persistent discrepancies between intake and expenditure are the key to changes in body weight and fat in adults.' In short, obesity in most people is caused by undramatic food excesses and just too little EXERCISE.

The point at which overweight becomes obesity is partly a judgement based on the patient's appearance, but in 1983 the Royal College of Physicians recommended acceptable weights according to the following table (*The Lancet*, 1 October 1983, p. 783):

	Men			Women		
Height without shoes (m)	Acceptable average	Acceptable range	Obese	Acceptable average	Acceptable range	Obese
1.45				46.0	42–53	64
1.48				46.5	42–54	65
1.50				47.0	43–55	66
1.52				48.5	44–57	68
1.54				49.5	44–58	70
1.56				50.4	45–58	70
1.58	55.8	51–64	77	51.3	46–59	71
1.60	57.6	52–65	78	52.6	48–61	73
1.62	58.6	53–66	79	54.0	49–62	74
1.64	59.6	54–67	80	55.4	50–64	77
1.66	60.6	55–69	83	56.8	51-65	78
1.68	61.7	56–71	85	58.1	52–66	79
1.70	63.5	58–73	88	60.0	53–67	80
1.72	65.0	59–74	89	61.3	55–69	83
1.74	66.5	60–75	90	62.6	56–70	84
1.76	68.0	62–77	92	64.0	58–72	86
1.78	69.4	64–79	95	65.3	59–74	89
1.80	71.0	65–80	96			
1.82	72.6	66–82	98			
1.84	74.2	67–84	101			
1.86	75.8	69–86	103			
1.88	77.6	71–88	106			
1.90	79.3	73–90	108			
1.92	81.0	75–93	112			
BMI	22.0	20.1–25.0	30.0	20.8	18.7–23.8	28.6

A similar table was published in the US in 1979. Note that according to these data, obesity is a weight up to 15kg more than the acceptable range for the height. Overweight, that is, weights between the acceptable range and obesity, is shockingly common in Britain. Among sixteen- to nineteen-year-olds, 15 per cent are overweight. Fifty-four per cent of men and 50 per cent of women aged sixty to sixty-five, more than a third of all adult men and just under a third of adult women are also overweight. It is even more disturbing to discover that the average weight for height of the population continues to rise.

Even mild overweight embodies a risk to health that is a matter for concern. For example, 'overweight children are very likely to become obese adults', said *The Lancet* in the report referred to above.

Familial tendencies to obesity appear to be primarily a result of parental pressure on children to eat. The tendency is not usually caused by genetic differences in METABOLISM, but reflects the self-image and sometimes the ignorance of the parents. The whole family tends to eat too much, often of the wrong foods.

Overweight and obese people are neither lazier nor more self-indulgent than people of average weight. They are either unaware of the risks, or they are unable to make the extra effort needed to get themselves in shape. Some overweight people may suffer from a psychological compulsion to eat too much in response to unhappiness or loneliness, but do not just as many people find that being lonely and unhappy destroys their appetites? Yet other overweight and obese people may be hysterical (see HYPNOTISM), but for most of us, perhaps the blame should fall on the universality of food advertising. We are made conscious of food as a social as well as a physiological necessity. One of the worst examples was a campaign by the dairy industry to sell us cream buns because they are 'naughty but nice'. If you are overweight, it is no exaggeration to say that cream buns can be life-threatening. The dangers fall into three categories. 1) The heart is forced to work too hard and may find the task impossible. 2) Diseases related to excessive fat intake include DIABETES, GALL STONES and degenerative disorders affecting the heart, arteries and kidneys. 3) Diseases caused by the adverse structural effects of too much weight. They include arthritis resulting from joint strain, hernia, varicose veins and even broken bones. Within reason, all three types of disease can be postponed if not completely avoided.

The best attack on obesity is diet and exercise. Without exercise, a low-calorie diet can also harm the arteries.

However, two NUTRIENTS cause the greatest number of problems: fats, especially saturated animal fats, and SUGAR. There is no need to suffer from an energy shortage just because you cut down on fats and sugar. Carbohydrate-containing food like BREAD, potatoes and pasta supply energy, and they supply other nutrients as well. Lean meats and vegetable OILS are probably better for you than fat meats and animal fats, but given a British or American diet, the more energy you obtain from CARBOHYDRATES (excluding sugar and ALCOHOL), the better. Sensible eating takes off weight and protects your health, but exercise within your strength and ability is equally essential.

There are undoubtedly obese people who cannot adhere to such a regimen, however. They may find a VERY LOW CALORIE DIET useful. In extreme cases, because of the dangers inherent in obesity, surgical removal of fat, dental splinting to make eating difficult and even a small balloon to fill the stomach may be prescribed.

See also DIET, BALANCED.

OIL

Liquid FAT from VEGETABLE seeds. Oil has the same ENERGY value weight-for-weight as animal fats such as butter and cream. It contains a higher proportion of polyunsaturated fatty acids (see LIPID) than animal fat and is the only food source of the essential fatty acid, linoleic acid. Oils contain no CHOLESTEROL. They are rich sources of VITAMIN E, and palm oil also contains a chemical which the body can convert to vitamin A.

Note that fish-liver oils are also liquid fats, but they are saturated. It is not usual to think of them as food, though they are used as dietary supplements to supply vitamin D.

Mineral oils such as paraffin are totally different chemical substances. They cannot be absorbed and pass through the digestive tract, acting as a laxative. Because they absorb vitamins A, D, E and K from the intestines, excessive use of mineral oil laxatives can lead to deficiencies of these vitamins.

Low-cholesterol diets include safflower, olive, sunflower,

SOYA, corn or peanut (groundnut) oil. Other vegetable oils such as cocoa butter and palm are relatively high in the saturated fatty acids, like animal fats, and are thought to contribute to the cholesterol synthesized by our bodies. Rape seed oil is a common constituent of mixed and cooking oils but should probably not be used in excess. Rape seed is a popular animal feed, and animals given large amounts develop heart damage.

The most widely-used vegetable oil is palm. Other important sources are corn, cotton seed, linseed, sesame, coconut and castor beans in addition to the more familiar types mentioned above. Cotton seed oil can contain a substance called gossypol, large amounts of which may be poisonous, though the evidence is contradictory. Castor oil contains ricinoleic acid, a fatty acid that irritates the intestinal lining. It is this irritation that produces its purgative effect.

The vitamin E in oils tends to delay rancidity because the vitamin slows OXIDATION. Nevertheless, light and warmth promote spoilage. Oil should always be stored in a dark, cool place. Spoilage and rancidity produce unpleasant changes of taste in oils, but they do not seem to be health risks.

OXIDATION-REDUCTION

Two aspects of a fundamental chemical process involved in the release of ENERGY from NUTRIENTS and in many other food-related events. For example, the process is a major cause of food spoilage.

Technically, oxidation is brought about by any one of three chemical changes, all three of which may occur at the same time: 1. addition of an oxygen atom to a compound; 2. removal of a hydrogen atom from the compound; 3. removal of one or more electrons from atoms in the compound. Reduction is the exact opposite: that is, removal of oxygen, addition of hydrogen or of electrons.

In an open system such as a lump of butter sitting on a dish in the larder, oxidation occurs through contact with the air. In a closed system such as a body cell, oxidation of one compound cannot occur without reduction of another one, and vice versa. Of course, it is true that oxidation of butter requires reduction of air, but air is a mixture rather than a chemical compound. In any case, this ubiquitous process is most familiar as the cause of rancidity which has nothing to do with spoilage caused by bacteria.

ANTIOXIDANTS are food ADDITIVES used to delay rancidity by preventing oxidation. VITAMIN E is a natural antioxidant though whether or not it acts in that role in the body is unclear. Conversely, vitamin C is an oxidizing agent: it promotes oxidation – and it does so in the body.

P

PHENTERMINE See DUROMINE

PHENYLALANINE

An AMINO ACID which cannot be made by the body in amounts necessary for health. Therefore, it must be obtained from food and is one of the eight essential amino acids.

Ironically, phenylalanine is also the only amino acid that may produce severe and lasting abnormalities because a few people suffer from a disease called phenylketonuria. Like other amino acids, phenylalanine is required for PROTEIN synthesis. A normal diet supplies adequate amounts, and excesses are broken down by an ENZYME and may be excreted. However, some infants lack the enzyme, an error caused because the necessary gene is missing or malfunctioning. Its absence may reflect either an inherited mistake or an inborn error. In any case, these children cannot break down phenylalanine. They develop slowly and display excessive irritability, but the most serious long-range effect is brain damage.

Fortunately, the disease can be identified early, and a diet containing carefully regulated amounts of phenylalanine will control the symptoms. The special diet will usually be maintained until the child is ten or twelve years old. It may then be safely discontinued but should be reintroduced during pregnancy to protect the foetus in the event that it has not inherited the mother's missing gene from the father.

Phenylalanine is also the chemical from which the body makes melanin, a pigment responsible for the colouring in hair and skin and for sun tanning. Another amino acid, tyrosine, is made from phenylalanine by body cells possessing the necessary gene.

PHOSPHORUS

A MINERAL used to form bones and teeth and in the process of ENERGY transfer and storage.

All foods excepting SUGAR contain phosphorus. It is usually associated with CALCIUM, and good sources of one will supply the other too. Exceptions are CEREALS, NUTS and PULSES in which the phosphorus is chemically part of a compound called phytic acid (see BREAD) which actually impairs calcium ABSORPTION. Because any reasonable diet supplies plenty of phosphorus, there is no recommended daily intake. However, if you are taking antacids regularly, you may need phosphorus supplements, because antacids prevent phosphorus absorption. The body will make up its needs by withdrawing phosphorus from bones which become weak and painful. Death will ensue if the drain is not stopped.

Most adults have between 600 and 900g (1–1½lb) of phosphorus in their bodies. Eighty to 85 per cent is in bones where it is combined with calcium to form apatite. Phosphorus is also a constituent of tooth dentine.

Its less visible functions are at least as significant as its structural role. With the expenditure of energy, phosphorus combines with oxygen to form phosphate. Up to three phosphates may be attached to a range of organic molecules such as the genetic molecule, DNA, and the several different molecules that store the energy obtained from the breakdown of CARBOHYDRATE. When stored energy is needed, for example, by muscles, the phosphates become detached and release their energy. Thus, the whole body economy depends on phosphorus.

In the form of phosphate, phosphorus is a common food ADDITIVE. It is used as an ANTICAKING AGENT and a SEQUESTRANT.

Both absorption and utilization of phosphorus, like that of calcium, depends on the presence of VITAMIN D and the HORMONE, parathormone. Excess phosphorus intake seems to be impossible. Either the mineral is not absorbed or it is excreted. On the other hand, phosphorus-containing tonics are of dubious value because the substance is so widely available in food. Most such tonics also contain ALCOHOL, however, and may therefore provide some pleasure and relaxation.

POISON, FOOD

'All substances are poisons: there is none that is not a poison: the right dose differentiates a poison and a remedy.' Thus wrote Paracelsus, a wise European physician who practised medicine almost 500 years ago.

Excess food, especially saturated FATS, causes overweight and may cause high blood pressure and heart disease. Excess food is undeniably poisonous. Similarly with many different foods. Too much chocolate can cause vomiting, constipation, skin disorders, headaches and other nervous conditions. ALCOHOL and WATER in excess are among the most obvious poisons.

As for poisons that may be found in food, there are two kinds: poisons that occur naturally and contaminants. Contaminants are either microbiological, TRACE ELEMENTS, pesticides or radioactive products.

Naturally-occurring poisons are found in plant food only. They are normally harmless because average portions contain very little. Of equal importance, these natural 'contaminants' are broken down in the course of normal metabolic (see METABOLISM) activity and do not accumulate in the body. Exceptions to these general statements are pointed out in the following list of familiar foods and the potentially-poisonous substances they normally contain:

Food	Poison	Comments
Almond	Oxalate, Linmarin	Linmarin becomes cyanic acid
Avocado	Amines	Pain if you also take MAO inhibitors (see CHEESE)
Banana	Amines	See Avocado
Beetroot	Oxalic acid	
Broad beans	Vicine	Can cause anaemia in those susceptible
Broccoli	Anti-iodine agents	Interfere with IODINE use causing goitre
Brussels sprouts	Anti-iodine agents	See Broccoli
Cabbage	Anti-iodine agents	See Broccoli
Cassava (TAPIOCA)	Linmarin	See Almond. Soaking and FERMENTATION required to prepare the root
Cauliflower	Anti-iodine agents	See Broccoli
Celery	Oxalic acid	
Cheese	Amines	See Avocado
Groundnut (peanut)	Trypsin inhibitors	Trypsin is a digestive ENZYME
Groundsel (some species)	Pyrrolizidine	Potentially cancer-causing
Kale	Anti-iodine agents	See Broccoli
Lima beans	Trypsin inhibitors	See Groundnut
Navy beans	Trypsin inhibitors	See Groundnut
Parsley	Oxalic acid	
Peas	Trypsin inhibitors	See Groundnut
Plantain	Serotonin	Possible cause of heart disease
Potato	Solanine	Could act like nerve gas. Concentration greater if potato turns green and if sprouting
	Safrole	Once used in US as FLAVOUR additive for BEER
Rhubarb	Oxalic acid	Leaves contain dangerous amounts. Immobilized by CALCIUM
SOYA BEANS	Anti-iodine agents	See Broccoli
	Trypsin inhibitors	See Groundnut
Spinach	Oxalic acid	
Sweet potato	Trypsin inhibitors	See Groundnut
Tea	Linmarin	See Almond
Tomato	Amines	See Avocado
Turnip	Anti-iodine agents	See Broccoli
Wheat	Gluten	Only affects those with COELIAC DISEASE
Wormwood	Thujone	Can cause convulsions. Used in absinthe and vermouth

Microbiological contaminants are bacteria, viruses, fungi,

moulds, worms or the toxins formed by these organisms. From the standpoint of numbers of people at risk, the most common of these microbiological contaminants, aflatoxin, is a toxin manufactured by a mould, *Aspergillus flavus*, which grows on improperly stored CEREALS and NUTS, especially groundnuts. Aflatoxin poisoning is rarely seen in Britain and America, but in the third world, notably in India where groundnut meal has become an important dietary supplement, it can be a nasty problem.

Probably the oldest known toxin, ergot, still causes occasional poisoning. It too is produced by a mould, *Claviceps purpurea*, especially on rye. Ergotism takes two forms, both potentially fatal: intense pain and possibly gangrene in the extremities, a disease once known in Europe as St Anthony's Fire, or cramps and convulsions. The chemical, ergot, has provided a foundation for the development of several clinically useful drugs and of LSD.

In the UK and the US, people who suffer the cramps, diarrhoea and vomiting symptomatic of acute food poisoning have most often succumbed to a bacterial infection by one of the Salmonellas. Many foods can become infected, but heat destroys the bacteria. Cooking must be thorough. It is salmonella in particular that is responsible for poisoning from frozen chicken or turkey which has not been completely thawed before it is roasted. However, cooked food left standing may also become infected by these common bacteria. They multiply if the food is reheated before serving. Therefore, food left to cool should be covered and refrigerated as soon as practicable. One reheating of a dish is usually the maximum that is safe.

About a third of the food poisoning cases in the UK are caused by a bacterium, *Clostridium welchii*, which is airborne and readily settles on food, especially joints of meat left uncovered for a long time. Again, reheating encourages bacterial growth. The rules applying to salmonella also fit Clostridium.

Although both salmonella and *Clostridium welchii* can kill the sick or elderly, by far the most dangerous bacterial cause of food poisoning is *Clostridium botulinum*. The disease is called botulism. The bacteria thrive in airless, acid-free foods such as tinned and bottled products. Nitrites are used as PRESERVATIVES to inhibit botulinus growth, and commercially canned food is heated to a high temperature to kill the bacteria. Home-bottled foods are a risk because temperature is less easily controlled. If the bacteria multiply during storage, they form a toxin chemically similar to nerve gas. Botulism is fatal in three-quarters of the cases that occur in Britain.

Although adequate cooking destroys most bacteria, it may not affect the toxins left behind by these organisms. For example, staphylococcus is a large family of common bacteria easily destroyed by heat, but their toxins which cause the symptoms of poisoning may persist. The answer is careful and continuous food hygiene.

1. Wash your hands before you prepare or eat any food.

2. Cooking surfaces, pots, pans and plates must be soap-and-water clean before every use.

3. Fresh FRUIT should be washed in cold water if it is not to be peeled, and should be stored in a refrigerator.

4. Uncooked VEGETABLES must be washed in cold water before preparation and kept in a refrigerator until they are eaten.

5. Cooked foods should be thoroughly cooked in accordance with the advice in any cookbook. Neither MEAT nor vegetables need to be cooked to death, but if meat was frozen, it must be completely defrosted before cooking. Pork is no more subject to spoilage than any other meat, and in Britain and America, the same rules apply to pork as to other cooked meat.

6. Food left to cool should be loosely covered against dust and refrigerated as soon as practicable.

7. Reheat cooked food no more than once. Refrigerate between uses.

8. If food looks or smells doubtful, throw it away – or return it to the shop where you bought it. Animals normally refuse bad food, and we have not totally lost the ability to judge what may have gone off. Trust your judgement. Do

not taste suspect food. A very small bite can contain enough of a toxin to make you ill.

9. Paring off moulds is no guarantee against infection because you can seldom see their tiny roots and tendrils. With CHEESE, however, mould or fungus often produces the desired texture and taste. Surface mould on cheese may be more unsightly and unpalatable than dangerous. If in doubt, though, throw the food away.

10. Place all waste in a separate bag or a container which is washed out regularly with soap and water. Remove waste from the kitchen as soon as it is practicable.

11. Store food either in a cool place or in a refrigerator, loosely covered.

12. Bear in mind that, antibiotics to the contrary notwithstanding, infectious organisms abound. In food, some of them can cause very unpleasant symptoms long before the doctor can get there.

If you or someone in your family develops cramps and starts vomiting, call the doctor. If you suspect food poisoning, the vomiting and even the diarrhoea should be encouraged – at least until the doctor gives instructions. Both symptoms are means of clearing the gut of the poison, at least in part. You must be sure, however, that the patient's fluids are kept up. If there is vomiting, this may not be easy. Sucking ice means that some fluid is being taken in, and the patient is less likely to vomit in response. Cold carbonated drinks like natural mineral water are more easily kept down than tap water. If the symptoms persist for more than six hours and a doctor is not available, you may also have to add small amounts of MINERALS, especially ordinary SALT, to the liquid. This is tricky and not ordinarily a first-aid measure, but packaged preparations are now available from chemists which do the job for you. Ask your doctor about them before the need arises.

Trace elements contaminating food are the familiar poisons of history and fiction: arsenic, mercury, lead and perhaps less well known, cadmium. The main sources of the first two are pesticides and industrial effluents. Pesticides can and always should be washed off food (see notes on hygiene, above). Mercury in sea water either from effluents or from rocks may be taken up by FISH or shellfish which then become poisonous. Constant safety checks in doubtful areas are now common practice. See also, radioactive products, below.

Lead contamination may be produced by industrial effluents, lead in cans and fumes from cars and factories. Washing removes surface deposits. The campaign against lead in motor fuel and your general awareness of the danger are the best general protections.

Cadmium contamination is caused in the same ways as lead contamination and affects shellfish. In the UK, the Bristol Channel is the only significantly polluted area.

In this context, it may be well to mention the dangers inherent in chemical additives in some animal food (see also MEAT). For example, until about 1950 a substance called diethylstilbesterol (DES) was added to livestock feed to encourage muscle growth. Its use was stopped when evidence mounted that DES caused cancer and birth defects. In the UK, animal food additives are now subject to testing and safety regulations analogous to those that apply to new drugs.

Pesticides and insecticides are ever more widely used to ensure the harvests needed to feed the growing world population. They are easily washed off food like apples that are eaten whole and uncooked. The difficulty really arises when sprayed vegetables or the chemicals on them are eaten by other species in what is known as the food chain. At the head of the chain, people eat the chemicals because they become part of the flesh of a fish, bird or mammal. Occasionally, chemicals from pesticides are even absorbed by plants through their roots. Many pesticides are not harmful to humans, but they may be metabolized (see METABOLISM) to poisons by other species in the food chain. So complex and unpredictable are the problems raised by adding chemicals to the environment that they are now being abandoned wherever possible. Scientists seeking to combat micro-organisms, worms and insects have turned to other solutions like genetic engineering designed to beat the organism at its own game. For example, a sterile insect pest may be introduced intentionally into an affected region so that within a generation, the pest population is at least halved. The side-effects of such measures on the ecosphere remain to be seen.

As to radioactive contamination, the problem grows as nuclear power stations multiply. Careless release of effluents into soil or water introduces radioactivity into the food chain where eventually it may affect humans. To fight the spread of nuclear power in a world desperately needing new energy sources is not only quixotic but downright stupid. (Obviously, this argument does not apply to the deadly and self-defeating spread of nuclear weapons.) Therefore, constant and intensive monitoring and regulation of waste disposal is the only answer at present. Leaks like those detected during 1983 at Sellafield in Cumbria must be prevented by all scientific means.

PONDERAX Ⓡ
An appetite suppressant available only on a doctor's prescription.

This drug was the first non-addictive appetite suppressant to be developed. It can cause mild side-effects such as headache, dizziness and sleep disturbances as well as loss of hair and, more seriously, anaemia – though the latter is rare. It should not be used by people suffering from depression, and those using it must not drink ALCOHOL.

The chemical name of Ponderax is fenfluramine hydrochloride. It is not an amphetamine like most of the earlier appetite suppressants (see APISATE, DUROMINE, TENUATE, TERONAC) and acts as a sedative rather than a stimulant.

POTASSIUM
A MINERAL required by the body if nerve and muscle cells are to function.

The average diet supplies ample potassium. Only FAT and SUGAR contain none. The richest sources are NUTS, wheat germ, dried FRUIT, instant COFFEE and BEER.

The adult body contains between 100 and 150g (3½–5oz)

of potassium. It is found primarily in the form of electri-
cally-charged atoms called ions which are needed to propa-
gate nerve signals and muscle contraction. Deficiencies are
rare, but diarrhoea and some drugs can cause severe
potassium loss. Symptoms of weakness and mental con-
fusion ensue. In extreme cases, kidney damage, a heart
attack and death can follow. The best antidote in most
cases is potassium-rich food.

POULTRY

Chicken, duck, goose, turkey. Because they are animals,
their flesh is MEAT.

Chicken and turkey contain less FAT on a weight for
weight basis than most cuts of beef, lamb and pork.
However, duck and goose are very fatty. The skin of all
poultry (and most other animals) is lined with a layer of
fat, and low-fat diets which often allow poultry interdict
the skin. Other NUTRIENTS in poultry are about the same as
in meat.

Frozen poultry is often full of WATER partly because of
the freezing process and partly because water has been
added intentionally to increase weight. It may be added
directly to the carcase, but water content can also be
increased by feeding the animal with certain chemicals.
Such practices are now controlled by law in the UK and
the US. For example, water uptake during freezing is
restricted to 7.4 per cent of weight.

Providing that the defrosting water is collected and used
for stock, frozen chicken should have the same nutrients as
fresh. In theory, they should also taste the same. Yet there
is little doubt that taste is affected both by freshness and by
the food the animal has been fed. Most people seem to be
able to tell the difference between the taste of a free-range
chicken and its battery-grown, frozen equivalent.

PREFIL ℝ

An appetite suppressant which acts by adding bulk to the
diet. However, the claim that Prefil suppresses appetite
lacks positive supporting evidence.

Providing enough fluid is drunk with it, Prefil is unlikely to be harmful. It can be bought at chemists without a doctor's prescription. Like other bulk fillers (see CELEVAC, CELLUCON, NILSTIM), it can produce flatulence and even bowel obstruction. Conversely, it may have a laxative effect. Allergy-like reactions have been reported in a few cases.

Prefil consists of sterculia, a powdered plant gum (see FIBRE).

PRESERVATIVE

A food ADDITIVE which delays or prevents spoilage due to microbial or ENZYME action.

Some thirty-four chemicals are permitted for use as preservatives in the UK, but several are similar to one another and, in fact, there are only thirteen basic compounds. The most commonly used is sulphur dioxide, followed by benzoic acid. Sodium nitrite and sodium nitrate are valuable especially for prevention of the growth of *Clostridium botulinum* which causes botulism, a frequently fatal form of food poisoning. Both of these sodium SALTS may be converted by the body into NITROSAMINES which are suspected carcinogens. NISIN is an antibiotic found naturally in some CHEESE and now used as a preservative.

Foods	Permitted preservatives
Bacon, ham, pickled MEAT	Sodium nitrite
Sausages, beefburgers, hamburgers	Sulphur dioxide
Raw potatoes, dehydrated VEGETABLES, dried FRUIT, jam	Sulphur dioxide
BEER, cider, WINE	Sulphur dioxide, Sorbic acid
SOFT DRINKS	Sulphur dioxide, Benzoic acid
Cheese	Nisin, Sorbic acid
BREAD	Propionic acid
Cakes, biscuits, pastry	Propionic acid, Sorbic acid
Canned food	Nisin

Early forms of food preservation such as salting, drying and smoking are still used, but smoke may be carcinogenic because it contains coal tar. SUGAR may be a preservative, as it is in jam. Acetic acid in VINEGAR and lactic acid in YOGHURT and sauerkraut are also natural preservatives.

Newer preservation technologies include dehydration and fast deep freezing, but both require sophisticated and expensive machinery.

PRITIKIN DIET

A high CARBOHYDRATE, very low FAT diet developed by a New York food writer, Nathan Pritikin. Also known as the Pritikin program.

Pritikin divides carbohydrates into high and low caloric density depending on the number of CALORIES per unit weight of food. High-caloric density carbohydrates include refined foods such as VEGETABLE OIL and SUGAR. FRUIT juices usually have a much higher caloric density than the fruits from which they come.

Low caloric density carbohydrates are CEREALS, FISH and MEAT, although the latter two are poor carbohydrate sources, and unprocessed foods containing other NUTRIENTS and FIBRE. Pritikin recommends a high fibre cereal for every breakfast, for example. Unfortunately for him, he failed to exploit the fibre aspect of his regimen, and the Pritikin program has been overtaken by a similar diet, the F-PLAN.

His menus are designed to provide 700, 850, 1000 or 1200 Calories a day for two weeks. The dieter selects the Calorie level most suitable for his or her needs. The menus are well balanced and tasty. For example, here are the respective dinners for day 5:

700 Calories: Salmon soufflé, cucumber-tomato salad, baked banana squash (a kind of courgette), raw vegetables.

850 Calories: As above, with more raw vegetables.

1000 Calories: As above, plus a water-based white sauce on the soufflé.

1200 Calories: As 1000 Calories, with two boiled potatoes as an alternative to the squash, and a dessert.

Pritikin quick fries in almost no oil in the Chinese manner to preserve VITAMINS. Sauces and dressings are made without fats. It is a sensible kind of diet with plenty

of bulk and variety. Unfortunately, it seems a little too
bland to hold the over-eater attracted to rich sauces or
cream buns. Yet there is no reason why FLAVOURS could
not be much more varied than his recipes and menus
suggest, especially in view of the Calorie-free spices that
are an integral part of Chinese-style quick frying. Beware
of soya sauce, however, because, as Pritikin points out, it
is very salty. Excessive SALT leads to water retention which
is neither good for your heart nor for weight loss.

PROCESSING, FOOD

Any preparation of food for consumption whether commercial or domestic, including brewing, cooking, freezing,
smoking and so on.

Food-processing is not twentieth-century technology.
Cooking must be assumed to have originated even before
the ability to control fire. Brewing and FERMENTATION have
been practised in every known civilization. Salting, smoking
and crop storage in cool cellars are ancient social inventions.
That the Chinese have milled rice throughout their long
history, moreover, is demonstrated by the discovery of
suitable implements dated to at least 8000 B.C. Indeed,
people in temperate climates have had to learn food processing in order to survive through the inter-harvest periods.

Sometimes the learning experience has been hazardous.
It is said of Francis Bacon, philosopher and alleged author
of Shakespeare's plays, that he was driving towards Highgate one snowy day when he wondered whether snow
might be used to preserve flesh. He and his companion
stopped the coach at the bottom of Highgate Hill, bought a
hen from a woman who lived nearby and stuffed the carcase
with snow. According to the story, Bacon caught a chill
that carried him off within a few days. What happened to
the hen was not recorded.

Broadly speaking, the techniques of food processing fall
under two headings: refining and preservation. Refining
includes flour milling, fermentation and the manufacture
of new products out of less edible natural foods; e.g.,

MARGARINE, SUGAR or TEXTURED VEGETABLE PROTEIN. Preservation is discussed under PRESERVATIVE.

Food processing may also be used to add natural or
artificial NUTRIENTS to food. Nutrients lost during processing can be added back, as is done when VITAMIN C is
added to dehydrated potatoes. CALCIUM, IODINE, IRON and
vitamins are added to white flour (see BREAD). Thus, adding
MILK to breakfast CEREAL is a kind of processing that adds
to the nutrients in both.

Domestic cooking is certainly the most familiar form of
food processing. Varied though cooking methods may
seem, they all serve one or more of three purposes.

1. To begin the breakdown of PROTEIN and soften the
tendinous protein capsules within which other nutrients
are held. All meat-cooking methods serve this purpose. It
applies also to cooking EGGS, although the effect of protein
breakdown is solidification.

2. To alter WATER content by adding or removing water
from the food. Baking bread removes water from the batter.
However, it also creates gases which cause the protein,
usually gluten, to stretch. To make pudding, you add water
to eggs and flour. Heating the pudding hardens the egg
protein as in 1, above. Some vegetables take on water when
they are boiled; for example, rice, but the actual cooking of
rice involves a third process.

3. Use of heat to break down CELLULOSE and other
indigestible CARBOHYDRATES, particularly in vegetables, so
that nutrients are more readily available for digestion. In
fact this process does for vegetables what 1, above does for
MEAT. Water may or may not be added. Thus, maize can
be heated and popped, or it can be boiled in water to make
it more easily digestible.

The art of cookery depends for its achievements in large
measure on the skill with which these processing steps are
carried out.

PROTEIN
The nitrogen-containing NUTRIENT required for growth and
repair and for the biosynthesis of all ENZYMES and many
HORMONES.

Most food provides some protein, but FRUIT offers very little, and there is no protein in FATS or SUGARS. The richest natural source is soya flour which is about half protein. EGGS, FISH, MEAT, most NUTS, POULTRY and dried PULSES including SOYA BEANS are excellent sources. MILK is mostly WATER, but dried skimmed milk contains roughly 35 per cent protein. About 10 per cent of the food content of CEREALS is protein. Other VEGETABLES offer less than half as much.

The body uses protein both structurally and functionally. The capsules surrounding limb muscles connect them to tendons, and the tendons themselves as well as the connective tissue are primarily protein. Nails and hair consist of protein plus some carbohydrate and pigments. Both cell membranes and the tiny structures inside cells consist of protein in part, but these proteins probably play functional rather than strictly structural roles.

Functionally, protein is omnipresent. As noted, all enzymes and many hormones are proteins. Some nonprotein factors also participate in the functions of these chemicals. Perhaps the most familiar example is the IRON at the heart of the protein haemoglobin molecule. The iron actually carries the oxygen, and it gives the colour to red blood cells. As enzymes, proteins also contribute to ENERGY creation, storage and use. Molecules similar in structure to haemoglobin inside all cells participate in energy creation and storage by facilitating the transmission of electron-sized units of energy from glucose sugar to storage molecules (see also PHOSPHORUS). Finally, protein is itself a source of energy, providing about 4 CALORIES per gram, the same as carbohydrates. Before it can be used for energy, however, protein must be converted to carbohydrate, an energy-consuming process. The nitrogen then becomes urea, a waste eliminated in the urine. In short, the biological use of protein for energy is highly uneconomic.

The fact that conversion of protein to fuel requires energy, however, underlies high-protein diets such as ATKINS, SCARSDALE and STILLMAN. By keeping fat and carbohydrate intake down, the body can be forced to draw on protein supplied in the diet. The energy conversion process is paid for out of fat stores. Apart from the minor disadvantages of these diets described in the respective entries, two more important problems must be faced: the first is that dependence on protein-breakdown for energy leads to a build up of KETONES in the blood. As a result, a tendency toward bad breath has often been remarked among high-protein dieters. Bad breath is not in itself a serious symptom, of course, but if ketosis is accompanied by continued disturbance of the ACID-base balance in body fluids, a threat to health exists (see also BASE, DIABETES).

The second important disadvantage of protein diets is more mundane: using protein to waste energy is a bit like using gold foil for cooking. The nitrogen needed to make protein can be incorporated into organic compounds only by certain vegetables which expend energy in the process. The nitrogen itself, on the other hand, cannot be used to make energy so the cost of its incorporation is lost. Nor are these costs imaginary sums in a cosmic energy balance. They are reflected in the fact that protein-containing food is expensive because it is relatively rare. Too often the world's poor, particularly those in tropical Africa, struggle to survive on a protein-deficient diet because they lack the power – that is, the energy – to pump water for irrigation or produce fertilizers (see KWASHIORKOR). A high-protein diet is inevitably an expensive diet.

The nitrogen atoms themselves are found in the AMINO ACIDS that become linked together to form proteins. Only about twenty amino acids make up the thousands of proteins with their myriad functions. Each protein consists of several hundred amino acids, and each protein has its peculiar structure determined by the chemical laws that govern the relationship of atoms in the amino acids. For example, the collagen in connective tissue consists of regularly repeating units which permit collagen to form long, straight chains. On the other hand, in haemoglobin two molecules of each of two different proteins, a total of four molecules, take up complex, connected conformations like four rubber bands rubbed together between the palms. In each haemoglobin molecule, the result of this protein structure is an opening that admits oxygen directly to the iron core, changing shape when oxygen is present and again when it is removed. Thus, each protein has a structure that determines its function. The sequence of amino acids that determines structure, moreover, is dictated by the genes inherited by every body cell (see ENZYME).

From the standpoint of nutritional needs, the measure of a protein's usefulness is the amino acids of which it is made. Our bodies can convert any amino acid into any other, but we lack the ability to make enough of eight amino acids. These eight are essential; that is, they are essential parts of the diet and must be obtained from food. Therefore, the nutritional quality of a protein depends on its content of the essential amino acids. In 1955, the Food and Agriculture Organization (FAO) of the United Nations proposed that the amounts of the essential amino acids needed be assumed to exist in an imaginary protein. This imaginary protein has become a reference against which protein quality can be measured, a sort of 100 per cent protein. The following foods are listed in order of their protein quality from high to low:

Eggs, cod, beef	100
Cheese	98
Cow's milk	95
Soya beans, polished rice, peanuts, peas, potatoes, whole wheat, corn	50 or less

Thus, the protein in eggs, for example, is of the highest quality despite the fact that there is more protein on a weight for weight basis in CHEESE and soya beans. GELATIN is pure protein, but it entirely lacks some essential amino acids. It is of a poor protein quality.

Clearly, the notion of protein quality is not merely academic. People whose diets consist of low-quality proteins must eat a lot more than those eating high-quality protein. It is now believed, moreover, that bulky, fibre-filled vegetables contribute benefits not obtainable from meat and similar high-quality, protein-containing foods. In affluent societies, people can afford to go on a high-protein diet including lots of expensive fish and lean meat, guaranteeing excessive intake of the essential amino acids. In poor regions where dietary choice is severely restricted, people depend on cassava or rice, foods containing low-quality proteins. Once again, the effect is MALNUTRITION, stunted development and even death.

About 20 per cent of body tissue by weight is protein. Not quite half of this is muscle. In adults, roughly 45g of protein must be replaced each day, though this quantity varies with body size and work done. Recommended daily protein intake is roughly twice this amount (90g), primarily because a diet with less protein tends to be so uninteresting. Children and pregnant women need relatively more. During illness and in times of emotional stress, furthermore, protein is often lost more rapidly and must be replaced. The following table shows a few of the foods common to the western diet and the amounts of protein contained in each:

Food (amount)	Protein (grams)
Baked beans, tinned (6oz)	about 10
Bread, wholemeal (4 thin slices)	10
Eggs, boiled (2 size 5)	25
Milk, whole (½ pint)	25
Mince (4oz)	27
TOTAL	about 92

PSYCHOLOGY, FOOD

Along with sex and protection against excessive heat or cold, hunger is a motivation which underlies the behaviour of every living organism, not least human behaviour. So fundamental is the drive for food that it is built into the brain. It could be argued that we must all eat because of physiological controls, but what and how much we eat and how we obtain our food is learned behaviour. This entry deals with the physiology and some of the learned aspects of food psychology. The significance of how food looks, tastes and smells is explored in entries on COLOUR and FLAVOUR. Psychologically-related disorders of eating are discussed in entries on ANOREXIA, BULIMIA and OBESITY.

The role of hysteria in eating behaviour is described briefly under HYPNOTISM.

Modern research has dissipated the notion of brain centres that regulate eating. Instead of well-defined groups of nerve cells, regulation is now thought to be the responsibility of tracts or sequences of cells in the brain with many connections that modify their activities. For example, given the present state of our knowledge about central control of appetite, the sensation of hunger could be reduced because of feelings of anxiety or fear. Suitable nervous connections needed to effect such interactions probably exist.

That is to say, nothing is as simple as it first appears, least of all the brain. Nevertheless, the appetitive tracts, formerly known as centres, are most evident in a part of the brain called the hypothalamus. Interestingly, the hypothalamus also contains nerve cells that affect anger, fear, sexual behaviour and emotions. There are two types of nerve cells affecting appetite. One is sensitive not only to nervous signals but also to the presence of glucose sugar in the blood. When blood sugar rises, as it does after a meal, these nerve cells signal satiety and the desire for food ceases. Another type of nerve cell operates independently of blood sugar and may control our perception that we are hungry. The two types of cells are probably interconnected and are certainly affected by what we have learned, such as, for example, good and bad smells. Incidentally, nerve cells in the hypothalamus which respond to the SALT concentration in body fluids regulate our sense of thirst. When salt concentration rises, we feel the need for water.

Everyone knows that eating slowly and chewing food thoroughly is a means of controlling appetite. It seems reasonable to assume that the actual physical work of eating signals the so-called satiety nerve cells that eating is going on. Or it may be that the stomach movements themselves, which do feed back signals to the brain, are given more time to deliver their message. These speculations indicate, however, that we do not know precisely why slow eating seems to reduce appetite.

On the other hand, chewing certainly gives more times

for ENZYMES in saliva to begin the DIGESTIVE PROCESS, and the gastric juices can work more rapidly on well-chewed bits than on lumps. Thus, deliberate eating probably improves digestion.

The nervous machinery regulating eating and drinking cannot explain the enormous range of gustatory behaviour that anyone can observe. Some people eat very much faster than others. Even within the same community, tastes differ markedly, and food choices are even more contrasting between different cultures. Some Chinese like flies. Some Americans consider rattlesnake a delicacy. Orthodox Jews will not eat shellfish, and neither Jews nor Muslims will eat pork. It may be true that anything not overtly poisonous which grows, walks, flies or swims will be eaten somewhere by someone, and rejected by someone somewhere else. In short, eating is very much learned behaviour.

One theory about how eating behaviour is learned – the stimulus-response theory central to behaviourism – underlies such regimens as the VAN ITALLIE CURE and WEIGHT WATCHERS. Other theories are possible. Thus, we could inherit more than the food-related nervous connections in the hypothalamus, though even these, it is important to realize, may be modified by our experiences. For example, taste buds respond only to a limited number of sensations: sweet, ACID, bitter and salt (see FLAVOUR). A preference for chocolate over coconut must be learned, but the fact that you can taste sugar but not haemoglobin, for example, means that your responses are determined in part by non-nervous inherited equipment. Baby monkeys seem to prefer a false teat that gives them milk if it is surrounded by soft carpet rather than by a wire frame. Is this in part learned, or almost wholly an inherited response?

Whatever eating entails in the way of machinery, learning about food is a fascinating and complex phenomenon. Watch an infant or a puppy experimenting. What they accept or reject is determined in part by the mother's behaviour. In the case of puppies, sibling behaviour may also play a role; they will compete for what the others in the litter also want. If a human mother indicates by grimaces that she doesn't like what the child is eating, the child may very well refuse to eat it too. If, on the other hand, she eats a little herself with evident pleasure, the child will be much more likely to eat.

It is easy to think of examples like this. Nor does the learning process stop suddenly at the age of four or six. Many of us discover that we have developed a taste for olives or for a vegetable that we once disliked, like spinach. Such changes in taste reflect our surroundings and the people we know, not a change in our nervous wiring or the shape of our taste buds. Yet the psychology of food, like all of our motivations, depends on both nature and nurture. New research is constantly shifting the emphasis between them, but to understand eating habits, both factors must be assigned their proper weight.

PULSES

1. A family of VEGETABLES including peanuts (groundnuts), peas and beans, also called legumes. 2. The edible seeds of legumes.

It is a mistake to think of pulses as just peas and beans. There are dozens of varieties of beans, each with its own FLAVOUR and culinary uses. French white beans, for example, are seldom sold in the UK or the US though they are available and make the superb sausage stew called cassoulet. It is cheap, filling and a good source of PROTEIN, ENERGY and FIBRE. Mange tout, the peas that are eaten pods and all, have slowly become more obtainable in London. SOYA BEANS are used not only on their own and to make soya flour, but also as a basis of artificial protein supplements to meat (see TEXTURED VEGETABLE PROTEIN). Many cooks think pulses are by far our most valuable and most underrated vegetables. They are better than average vegetable sources of protein and the B VITAMINS, especially B_1 and B_2. They also contain vitamins A and C, CARBO-HYDRATE, much of it in the form of indigestible FIBRE, and they are good sources of energy. Only soya beans contain FAT. Soya is also rich in IRON, but all pulses provide some MINERALS. An average portion of baked beans contains about the same protein as an EGG, but the protein quality is lower; that is, bean protein is low in the essential AMINO ACID, methionine. It supplies the body's needs less adequately than egg protein.

Freezing and canning fresh pulses can preserve their B vitamins and only slightly reduces other vitamin content. However, losses do occur during storage, defrosting and cooking. Dried pulses retain their protein, carbohydrate and vitamin B_1, but other vitamins are largely lost in the drying process. Vitamin C is most abundant when dried pulses have just begun to sprout.

R

RHEUMATISM DIET

On the theory that at least one cause of rheumatism is the food we eat, the notion of a diet that can control if not cure the disease emerged. It is an old notion but, unfortunately, it still lacks objective scientific proof.

Rheumatism diets vary with the authority and the underlying theory about what foods are involved. One modern health encyclopedia recommends that wholewheat BREAD should replace white, all white SUGAR should be avoided and supplements of vitamins C, D and E should be taken. Clearly, this regimen could not have been recommended before vitamins were identified early this century, nor does it recognize modern medical advice that brown sugar is no better for you than white.

Rheumatism is an imprecise term covering symptoms ranging from an aching joint to the pain and swelling more properly designated arthritis. In some people, some symptoms may be due to improper diet. For example, this may be the case with overweight people whose muscles and joints are overstressed. Some symptoms of rheumatism may even be due to food ALLERGY. Only detailed medical tests can identify the causes of a symptom and provide a possible foundation for cure.

S

SACCHARIN

A SWEETENER and sugar-substitute. Although it was not introduced until the SUGAR shortage imposed by World War I, saccharin was discovered accidentally in 1879. In English, the word is now a synonym for sweet.

A simple chemical, closely related to the famous sulpha drugs, the first antibiotics, saccharin contains no CALORIES. It is 300 times as sweet as sugar. Such figures are derived from taste tests in which a large number of subjects are asked to taste solutions of both sugar and saccharin. The solutions are made progressively more dilute until the subject fails to taste anything. It was found that a saccharin solution could become 300 times more dilute than a sugar solution before most subjects ceased tasting it.

Eaten alone, saccharin leaves a bitter after-taste. During the 1960s, massive doses were shown to cause cancer in laboratory animals. The risk to human users from the amounts needed in COFFEE or TEA is so low, however, that saccharin is permitted by all governments.

SALT

1. Table or cooking salt. 2. A compound formed by chemical combination of an ACID with a BASE. The most familiar example is SODIUM plus hydrochloric acid which produces WATER plus sodium chloride.

All FRUIT, MEAT and VEGETABLES contain some salt because both the sodium and the CHLORINE are needed by living tissue. For example, nerves and muscles could not function without both elements. A normal diet including salt added in cooking provides about 10g a day and adding salt before eating can double that amount. Most of us cannot use that much salt. Some is excreted, but the sodium and chloride that is held by the tissues tends to attract water by osmosis. Osmosis is a physical process causing the relative amounts of water and substances dissolved or emulsified in water to balance on both sides of blood-vessel walls. More salt in the tissues draws more water from the blood which must then be replaced by drinking. Everyons knows that the more salty the food, the more you want to drink.

Thus, any slimming diet will begin by cutting down salt intake and keeping it down. The dieter may be surprised by how quickly taste changes. It is relatively easy to reduce your appetite for salt. Much of the salt in our diets is put there by food processors (see PROCESSING, FOOD), but there is much we can do ourselves to reduce salt intake. For example, you should never salt meat before cooking it. Health reasons aside, added surface salt toughens meat. Note the effect of salt on pork crackling. Many bottled sauces, moreover, are extremely salty.

Although reducing salt intake can help to control weight, health or so-called slimming salts can no longer be sold. Glauber's or EPSOM SALTS will certainly remove water from your body because it is a purgative which produces diarrhoea. Such loss is fugitive and artificial if not downright harmful. As to slimming salts added to the bath water, the idea is so silly that it is hard to believe anyone ever took it seriously.

SCARSDALE MEDICAL DIET

A high-protein, low-carbohydrate, low-fat diet named for the suburban New York town where it was originated by Dr Herman Tarnower.

In this regimen, PROTEIN rises from about 10 to 15 per cent of total food intake to about 43 per cent. SUGAR is absolutely prohibited, but raw VEGETABLES and fat-free liquids such as black COFFEE or TEA may be taken *ad libitum*. Other foods are rigidly controlled. The actual reduction in food quantity depends on the dieter, but everyone is required to reduce FAT intake by approximately half to roughly 25 per cent of daily food intake. This figure would be warmly welcomed by recent official dietary studies in the UK (see DIET, BALANCED). The principal attack on CARBOHYDRATES in the Scarsdale diet is elimination of sugar and sweets, pasta, potatoes and all BREAD excepting a 'high-protein' product based on wholemeal flour. ALCOHOL is permitted in very small amounts only during the bi-monthly relief periods from the rigidly fixed diet.

This two-stage approach to weight loss is the special feature of the Scarsdale diet. For the first two weeks, the dieter is confined to an absolutely fixed regimen, the Medical Diet, without alcohol, sugar, OILS or fat MEATS. For example, the skin must be removed from chicken before it is eaten. Naturally, the dieter will experience a satisfying weight loss. During the next two weeks, he or she moves from the Medical Diet to a Keep-Trim Program. Keeping Trim allows some limited relief in the form of a small daily alcohol allowance and sugarless and fat-free sweets, the kind usually sold for diabetic diets. Nor is the dieter restricted to specified dishes for each meal. He or she may select freely from the list of permitted foods.

If the dieter sticks to the permitted foods and if the quantities don't rise unreasonably, he or she should continue to lose weight. The author seems not to have expected these conditions to be met during the Keep-Trim Program, however, because he says that during this second fortnight, weight loss will all but stop. Therefore, during the next two weeks, the dieter returns to the Medical Diet, and so on through fortnightly alternations until the target weight loss is reached. Thereafter, and for the rest of the dieter's life, he or she must adhere to the Keep-Trim Program.

This two-phase schedule has a medical as well as a psychological objective. The very high protein Medical Diet will produce excess KETONES with a resulting ketosis that can become dangerous if it is allowed to continue (see also PROTEIN). Although protein-containing foods are still important in the Keep-Trim Program, that Program allows a more balanced diet to be achieved. Incidentally, it is worth noting that the author expects the dieter, left to his or her own devices, to return without being told how to a more healthful normal diet.

One of Tarnower's aims was to evolve a diet programme that would have the support and cooperation of his fellow medical professionals. He used two other simple, medically acceptable techniques to attract dieters. They are given the task of having regular weight checks, especially during the Keep-Trim periods and later after they have achieved their target weights. Second, Tarnower encourages dieters to look at the positive side of their dieting. He urges that they think about what they can eat rather than what is forbidden. He encourages experiments with HERBS and spices to enhance the variety of the food, and he stresses the importance of how food looks on a plate. Even if the dieter is eating alone, meals should be attractively presented. The dieter is then encouraged to eat slowly and to chew thoroughly, the oldest and most sensible instructions on how to obtain satisfaction out of what you eat.

Apart from its potential health hazards, the Scarsdale Medical Diet has one other obvious problem: it can be expensive. The cost of lean chops and steaks may have been relatively unimportant to Tarnower's well-healed Scarsdale patients, but he wrote his book for mass consumption. Money-saver principles had to be introduced. They include soya-based meat substitutes and the VEGETARIAN Scarsdale diet. Note, however, that meat substitutes are usually TEXTURED VEGETABLE PROTEIN (TVP) which can add a new health risk to the diet. TVP lacks essential AMINO ACIDS which the dieter must obtain from other sources such as meat or YEAST.

SEQUESTRANT

A food ADDITIVE intended to prevent VITAMIN destruction and food spoilage. Sequestering agents may also be called chelating agents.

Some TRACE ELEMENTS, especially the metals IRON and copper, have no adverse effects on fresh food, but in processed products they cause loss of NUTRIENTS, discolouration and other forms of spoilage. For example, vitamins A, B$_1$, folic acid, C and E are lost in the presence of iron or copper. They contribute to the rancidity of FATS and cause clouding of SOFT DRINKS and BEER.

A sequestrant combines with trace elements such as these

MINERALS and prevents their adverse effects. Sequestrants serve a similar purpose to ANTIOXIDANTS, but their chemical role is more restricted.

The most common sequestrant is a synthetic compound called ethylenediamine tetraacetic acid, EDTA. Others commonly used are organic compounds such as phosphates (see PHOSPHORUS), citric acid (see ENERGY), tartaric acid and the SALTS of the latter two. An AMINO ACID, glycine, found in all body PROTEINS is also permitted in the UK, but it is not on the FAO/WHO list of approved sequestrants.

These substances work because their molecules form a kind of cage which captures and immobilizes the metal atom. The process is properly called metal chelation. However, it must be recognized that the trace elements in foods containing sequestrants are no longer available as nutrients.

SLENDER ®

A SLIMMING AID, but a food, not a drug. One sachet is the basis for a complete meal. Each sachet consists of sweetened dried skimmed MILK plus small quantities of other ingredients. It is to be mixed into one-third of a pint of milk. The combination contains 229 CALORIES. Thus, Slender can be used as a VERY LOW CALORIE DIET (see also COMPLAN).

In addition to CARBOHYDRATE, FAT and PROTEIN, Slender has CALCIUM, IODINE, IRON and VITAMINS A, B_1, B_2, B_3, B_6, C, D and E.

SLIMMING AID

A product intended to reduce the desire for food. Slimming aids fall into four categories: SUGAR substitutes, bulk fillers, drugs and low-calorie foods.

Sugar substitutes are artificial SWEETENERS such as ASPARTAME and SACCHARIN. They may be used by a dieter who cannot drink COFFEE or TEA unless it is sweetened.

Bulk fillers include CELEVAC, CELLUCON, NILSTIM and PREFIL. These products add bulk in the stomach on the theory that the dieter will then feel full. There is no consistent experimental evidence to support these claims, perhaps because the bulk fillers do not reduce the psychological wish for certain foods: for example, cream buns or chips. They are fairly harmless substances but can produce gas, distension and both diarrhoea and constipation depending on what else is eaten.

Slimming drugs all act by suppressing the wish for food. In other words, they affect the brain. The first drug used to suppress appetite was amphetamine, a compound that is addictive and now rarely prescribed. APISATE, DUROMINE, and TENUATE (or Ionamin) are amphetamine-like drugs with a number of undesirable side-effects including the possibility of addiction (see also TERONAC). An entirely different compound, PONDERAX, is probably not addictive though it does have side-effects. All of these drugs share one disadvantage. After periods that vary with the user and the drug, they stop working. Despite the drug, the dieter feels hungry. This discouraging course of events reflects the fact that all drugs are foreign to the body: they are potentially poisonous. ENZYMES, especially in the liver, break down drugs, but it often takes time for the body to synthesize enough of an enzyme to detoxify a previously unfamiliar drug. Thus, the period during which the appetite suppressant works varies. A similar loss of effectiveness due to the development of tolerance affects many drugs used to treat real illnesses.

THYROID hormones are sometimes used to control weight but only under direct medical supervision. The HORMONES increase METABOLISM with a risk of damage to the heart and kidneys.

In 1984, a new kind of slimming drug was tested. It was designed to increase the body's utilization of brown fat on the theory that this process slightly increases metabolism (see FAT). Whether a pill with such widespread effects on body chemistry will prove to be safe remains to be seen. (See also STARCH BLOCKER.)

Low-calorie foods are expensive but perhaps not always useless slimming aids. Beware of low-calorie BREAD, however. The calorie content is exactly the same as that of

ordinary bread, but the slice is smaller and costs proportionately more. Diet SOUPS, SOFT DRINKS and sweets usually
contain fewer CALORIES than ordinary equivalents. Sugar
substitutes are used in their manufacture, and low-calorie
soups use synthetic THICKENERS instead of cornstarch or
flour. AYDS, BRAN-SLIM, COMPLAN, ENERGEN, GLUCODIN,
SLENDER and TRIOSORBON are available without prescrip-
tions through chemists and some food chains. They are
foods rather than drugs. Their contents vary, but they
share a problem: they cannot indefinitely control appetite
simply because the boredom factor applies to them just as
it does to raw VEGETABLES and fresh FRUIT.

SODIUM
A MINERAL required for bone growth, normal operation of
nerves and muscles and to regulate the amount of WATER in
the body.

Most sodium is absorbed in the form of SALT, sodium
chloride. However, animal products such as EGGS, FISH,
MEAT and MILK contribute small amounts of pure sodium.
Bicarbonate of soda and baking powder also contain
sodium.

If excessive sweating causes a severe loss of sodium
which is not immediately replaced, the body dehydrates.
Water is lost with the sodium in order to maintain the
normal balance between minerals and water. Extreme
fatigue, headache and weakness will be followed by convulsions, coma and death unless the sodium deficit is
quickly made up.

Like hydrogen, sodium exists in the body as a positively-
charged ion. It is directly responsible for the electrochemi-
cal signals sent by nerve cells and for the contraction of
muscles. As a major source of positive electrical charge,
moreover, sodium affects the ACID-base balance of the body
fluids (see BASE).

The body contains between 75 and 100g (3–3½oz) of
sodium, 90 per cent of it dissolved in body fluids. The
average diet adds between 4 and 8g per day most of which

is eliminated in the urine, but a loss of more than 8g can produce the danger signs of dehydration.

SOFT DRINKS

Non-alcoholic beverages customarily excluding COFFEE, MILK, TEA and WATER. Soft drinks fall into two categories: FRUIT juices and artificial beverages including low-calorie drinks.

Citrus fruit juices have been recognized as pleasant sources of VITAMIN C for many years and as refreshing drinks throughout history. A glass of freshly-squeezed orange juice in the morning is a marvellous pick-me-up as well as a means of enhancing the ABSORPTION of IRON from EGGS and toast. All citrus fruits contain citric acid which helps to retain vitamin C. Stored in tightly-closed jars, cans or bottles, the vitamin is retained fairly well, but OXIDATION rapidly reduces it when it comes into contact with air. For that reason, citrus fruit juices in waxed boxes lose vitamin C from the moment they are opened.

Blackcurrant juice is also a rich source of vitamin C, but natural apple juice contains very little. All the fruit juices have small amounts of SUGAR and make good supplements for low-calorie diets. For many people, apple juice is an acceptable substitute for BEER or WINE with meals.

Artificial beverages are a different matter. Their main ingredients are water and sugar or a sugar substitute. Other NUTRIENTS such as vitamins may be added along with COLOUR and FLAVOUR. As with other packaged foods, the labels must list all ingredients of these drinks.

Fruit-'flavoured' drinks and '-ades' contain no fruit. Squashes, crushes and cordials must be made with legally specified amounts of the named fruits, but they are low. Drinks 'made from whole fresh' fruits, that is comminuted drinks, may contain even less fruit than squashes.

Cola drinks consist of CAFFEINE, phosphoric acid, carbon dioxide for the bubbles, flavourings, colour (usually caramel) and sugar, Lucozade ® and other glucose drinks replace sucrose, the most familiar form of sugar, with glucose which is less sweet. Tonic water, bitter orange and bitter lemon usually obtain their flavours from small quantities of quinine, the ancient cure for malaria. They also contain carbon dioxide.

Low-calorie drinks must have no more than 1½ C per fluid ounce. This is easy to achieve because with the exception of water the ingredients are synthetic and nutrient-free as well as calorie-free.

SOUP

Conventionally, a meat-, fish- or poultry-based stock which may contain CEREAL, FRUIT and VEGETABLES. In practice, the stock may be made from the food contents themselves or from synthetic MEAT flavours. Meat is not a necessary constituent.

Obviously, the nutritional value of the soup depends on what is in it. Meat stock is WATER plus some FAT, MINERALS, PROTEIN and, if the water was used first to boil green vegetables, some B VITAMINS. Clear soups are practically Calorie-free and are recommended for weight control. Thick soups are those with pureed vegetables or other THICKENERS. They may also contain MILK or cream as last-minute additions. If they do, their CALORIE content is enhanced accordingly. 'Creamed' canned soups contain thickeners and some cream or butter fat, however. Like clear soup, broth has little NUTRIENT value though some people may find that it stimulates appetite.

Commercial tinned soups but not instant soups have about the same nutrients as homemade soup. Cornstarch adds a few calories when it is used for thickening, but the common synthetic thickeners do not. There is a UK Code of Practice affecting soups which does not have the force of law. Under it:

1. Meat soups must contain a minimum of 6 per cent meat and Scotch broth a minimum of 3 per cent.

2. Unless otherwise stated, consommé must be made from meat stock.

3. In vegetable soups, a single-vegetable soup like tomato should contain more tomato than any other vegetable.

Mixed vegetable soup should have at least four vegetables. Green pea soup should be made from fresh or frozen peas.

4. Cream soups must contain butter fat.

Packaged, dehydrated soups are unregulated, but the contents must be listed on the package. Many instant soups are entirely synthetic with the exception of the milk or water you add and contain no nutrients and no Calories.

SOYA BEAN

(*Glycine max*) A PULSE. It originated in the Far East and is still an important crop there. However, the largest producer today is the US. The plant requires a hot summer and is susceptible to frost.

Soya beans contain more PROTEIN weight for weight than any other substance, between 40 and 50 per cent. Unfortunately, soya protein lacks one of the essential AMINO ACIDS, methionine, and cannot support life alone, at least in theory. The fact is that the body does make small amounts of all essential amino acids. In the face of total deprivation and in the absence of unusual demands, some adaptation appears to take place. Neither soya nor any other VEGETABLE protein will suffice during pregnancy or the rapid growth of childhood, however.

About 22 per cent of soya beans are FAT and the beans provide more OIL than any other source. It is polyunsaturated and thought to be less damaging to the heart and blood vessels than animal fats (see LIPID).

Soya now feeds millions of people as soya bean concentrate or more commonly as soya protein concentrate. It is the principal constituent of TEXTURED VEGETABLE PROTEIN, a MEAT substitute used in many processed foods.

SPIRITS

Beverages containing concentrated ALCOHOL such as whisky, gin, vodka, brandy and liqueur. In Britain, spirits must be at least 65 degrees proof (see ALCOHOL). Liqueurs contain more alcohol than any other spirituous drink.

Spirits can be made from any fermented CARBOHYDRATE. Whisky and gin are made from CEREALS, vodka and rye whisky from potatoes, liqueurs from the FRUIT usually specified in the name such as oranges, cherries or cocoa beans. In each case, the ferment is distilled to drive off WATER. FLAVOURS come from the original ferment. They may also be added during DISTILLATION as juniper berries and coriander are added to gin, or they may be synthetic.

STABILIZER

A food ADDITIVE which helps to maintain an emulsion when it has been formed. They are widely used, especially in commercial BREAD production, pastries, ice-cream, MAR-GARINE, chocolate and other sweets.

An emulsion is a mixture of two substances like OIL and WATER which are not soluble in each other. Mayonnaise is an emulsion of oil and VINEGAR (which is mostly water) given a long life by the inclusion of EGG yolks as EMULSI-FIERS. Stabilizers may work like emulsifiers, but the most common are gums which increase the viscosity or thicken one of the constituents. Gums are indigestible plant CARBO-HYDRATES such as gum arabic, agar, carageenan and pectin. Chicle, the basis of chewing-gum, is a non-carbohydrate plant gum and cannot act as a stabilizer. Gums have unexpected stabilizing properties. For example, they help to hold the foam on a pint of BEER. By binding excess water, they reduce ice crystal formation in ice-cream. Increased thickness in mayonnaise or MILK-shakes imparted by a stabilizer is thought to improve palatability.

See also THICKENER.

STARCH

A major food source of CARBOHYDRATE. Plants store the SUGAR, glucose, as starch. It does not exist in animals.

TAPIOCA, sago, arrowroot and cornflour are almost pure starch. CEREALS contain up to 70 per cent by weight. Potatoes are about 20 per cent starch and the PULSES between 10 and 15 per cent. Starch is mixed with VITAMINS, MINERALS and FIBRE in all of these sources excepting the first four. BREAD, NUTS and root VEGETABLES also contain some starch in combination with other NUTRIENTS.

Cereals, potatoes and pulses are among the most useful sources of ENERGY. Fashionable attitudes and low-carbohydrate diets overlook the value of starchy foods that provide energy mixed with other nutrients. Even the low-carbohydrate diets prescribed for diabetics (see DIABETES) include starchy foods in controlled amounts. Refined carbohydrates such as SUGAR contain few other nutrients and no fibre. They are unnecessary no matter how tempting. Similarly, people worried about their weight can cut CALORIES by reducing their intake of OIL and FAT, especially animal fat. For the normally healthy person, however, bread and boiled or baked potatoes with a little butter, MARGARINE or, even better, YOGHURT are sensible parts of a balanced diet.

Starch consists of a long chain of linked glucose molecules. GLYCOGEN, so-called animal starch, is also a linked chain of glucose molecules, but the nature of the links in the two carbohydrates differs. Starch yields the same energy as glucose, 4 C per g. Because of its molecular structure, it dissolves only slowly in water. Heating hastens the process, one of the reasons for heating sauces thickened with flour or cornstarch. Standing also allows time for starch to dissolve as when a batter stands before use.

During digestion, the starch molecule breaks down into its constituent glucose molecules. The process begins in the mouth with the action of a salivary ENZYME, amylase. Thus, chewing bread or potatoes thoroughly produces a sweetish taste. Glucose is quickly absorbed through the small intestine. See also ABSORPTION, DIGESTIVE PROCESS. It may be withdrawn from the blood for immediate use or stored in the form of glycogen.

STARCH BLOCKER

A drug designed to prevent digestive breakdown of STARCH so that it cannot be absorbed into the body. Thus, it was intended as a SLIMMING AID, but all such claims have been proven false.

STERCULIA See PREFIL

STILLMAN DIET

A high-protein diet developed by Dr Irwin M. Stillman, a New York physician. Stillman recommended the diet for people with arthritis in the hope that if they reduced their weight, the pain from their swollen joints would be helped either directly or indirectly (see RHEUMATISM DIET).

The Stillman diet increases the intake of B VITAMINS though the benefits to be expected are unclear. It reduces SODIUM intake because low-salt diets help to reduce the amount of WATER in the body and help to keep weight down. Under the Stillman regimen, the risk of ketosis (see KETONE), especially in older people immobilized by arthritis, is just as great as it is with any other high-protein diet (see ATKINS, PROTEIN, SCARSDALE).

SUGAR

Pure CARBOHYDRATE. Common white sugar is sucrose. Other sugars in food include glucose (MEAT and FISH), fructose (FRUIT), maltose (BEER and liqueurs) and lactose (MILK). All sugars produce 4.1 CALORIES per gram. Fructose is the sweetest, almost twice as sweet as sucrose. Lactose is the least sweet, only one-fifth as sweet as sucrose. For a description of the tests on which such judgements are based, see SACCHARIN.

Sucrose comes primarily from sugar cane and sugar beet. Demerara is also refined from cane but retains some of the raw sugar COLOUR. Other brown sugars are mixtures of refined sugar and syrup dried to form crystals. Although there are traces of MINERALS in demerara and brown sugar, they too are practically pure carbohydrate and no better for you than white sugar. Consumption of a teaspoonful of sugar, about 10g, provides about 40 calories with no other nutritional benefit. Other carbohydrates such as the STARCH in BREAD provide energy at the same rate, but the carbohydrate is mixed with FIBRE, minerals, PROTEIN and VITAMINS. Bread and potatoes are carbohydrate-rich foods which contribute additional NUTRIENTS and fibre to a balanced diet. Sugar is called empty carbohydrate.

Sugar consumption is directly implicated in tooth decay.

This relationship holds also for brown sugar and for HONEY. Sugar and honey provide a medium or food on which the major bacterial cause of tooth decay, *Streptococcus mutans*, thrives. This bacterium produces ACIDS that dissolve tooth enamel; it also converts sugar to a kind of glue which attaches the bacteria to the teeth and gums, and it makes saliva a less effective antidote to destructive acids than it normally is. Sugar actually increases the level of acid in the mouth exacerbating the loss of tooth enamel. Every time you eat or drink sugar, your mouth becomes more acid. If you take sugar three or four times a day, the acidity remains fixed at a level that dissolves enamel faster than the body can replace it. By the same token, enamel reconstruction will occur if you refrain from sugar and allow the saliva to reduce the acidity in your mouth. Enamel restoration is enhanced by the presence of fluoride in WATER and tooth paste (see FLUORINE). However, neither fluoridation nor regular tooth brushing with fluoride toothpastes will prevent tooth decay if the amount of sugar you eat remains high, and especially if you continue to take sugar at regular intervals throughout the day.

In the UK and the US, a safe level of sugar consumption is considered to be no more than 15kg (roughly 33lb) per year (see DIET, BALANCED). This amounts to about half a pound a week or three teaspoonfuls a day. That may sound a lot, and it is, but bear in mind that it includes the sugar in food, jam, sweets, pastries, SOFT DRINKS and BEER. The kind of sugar or its source do not effect its adverse actions. At present, moreover, the average sugar consumption in the UK is 38kg per year, not 15!

Molasses, treacle, golden syrup and corn syrup contain slightly fewer Calories than sugar, but their effect on tooth decay is the same. Molasses remains when sugar has been crystallized out of cane or beet juice. Treacle and golden syrup are refined from molasses. Corn syrup is pure glucose made from STARCH, usually corn starch.

Sucrose, maltose and lactose each consist of two sugar molecules combined. Sucrose consists of glucose plus fructose, maltose of two glucose molecules and lactose of glucose plus galactose. The two sugars are split apart during digestion and the single sugars are absorbed. Glucose can, of course, be converted directly to ENERGY, but fructose and galactose must be converted to glucose by ENZYMES principally in the liver.

SULPHUR

An element required to make certain AMINO ACIDS, the HORMONE insulin (see DIABETES) and antibodies (see ALLERGY, FOOD).

Most of the sulphur in food is part of PROTEIN which contains the sulphur-bearing amino acids, methionine and cysteine. Methionine is also one of the essential amino acids. Cysteine and a similar amino acid, cystine, can be synthesized by the body in adequate amounts providing sulphur is available. Both insulin and antibodies require sulphur to act as atomic links holding together large segments of the respective molecules. The VITAMINS thiamin, B_1, and biotin also contain sulphur.

In the form of sulphur dioxide, sulphur is a PRESERVATIVE and may be added to many foods.

SWEETENER

A food ADDITIVE intended to give a sweet taste. The most common and familiar is sucrose, ordinary white SUGAR.

Synthetic sweeteners such as ASPARTAME and SACCHARIN are much sweeter than sugar and contain no CALORIES. Cyclamate was a popular sweetener for many years, but it is now suspected of being a cancer-causing chemical.

Synthetics are useful for diabetic diets and to FLAVOUR low-calorie drinks and desserts. However, there are disadvantages. Some synthetics leave an unpleasant aftertaste. Under biological conditions, they may become unstable and lose their sweetness. Unlike sugar, moreover, there may be a time-lag between tasting the sweetener and the onset of a sense of sweetness. This characteristic could be useful in chewing-gum where the flavour should last, but it is not acceptable in food and drink.

Sucrose has none of these faults, and it is both natural

and cheap. It also thickens watery solutions, has limited
PRESERVATIVE qualities and can be used to create glacés,
functions which none of the artificial sweeteners can perform. Its drawbacks are examined in the entry on SUGAR.

The problem confronting scientists looking for better
synthetic sweeteners is our very limited understanding of
the sense of taste (see FLAVOUR). All the existing synthetics
have actually been found by accident. Two other interesting
substances are now being studied: maltol, a synthetic, has
no taste itself but enhances sweet or fruity tastes in a
manner analogous to the way MONOSODIUM GLUTAMATE
enhances MEAT flavours; miraculin, obtained from the
berry, *Richardella dulcifera*, causes sour substances to taste
sweet if it is applied directly to the tongue first.

T

TAPIOCA

The Asian name for cassava or manioc. The plant is
Manihot utilissima. After preparation of the tubers from
which tapioca comes, the edible flakes or pearls are milled
into flour to make garri in Nigeria and farinka in Brazil.

The plant is easy to grow, and storage is simple because
many varieties can be left in the ground for long periods
before they are used. Being largely starch, tapioca is almost
pure CARBOHYDRATE. Like SUGAR, it contributes practically
no other NUTRIENTS to the diet unless it is cooked with
other foods such as MILK. Yet in parts of Nigeria, for
example, tapioca is the only food naturally available. The
result is that KWASHIORKOR is widespread.

Before tapioca is milled, the tubers must go through a
process of FERMENTATION and heating. In this way, the
cyanide contained in the tubers is broken down.

TEA

Second only to WATER as the world's most popular beverage. It is made from the leaves of one of two species of
tree, *Camellia thea* or *Thea sinensis*. Tea-drinking originated

in China as early as 3000 B.C. It first reached England and
probably Europe in 1657.

Tea contains about 50 to 80mg of CAFFEINE per cup,
about half the amount in COFFEE, but it also has a related
drug, theophylline, which is a stimulant like caffeine. There
are traces of FLUORINE, manganese, VITAMINS B₂ and B₃
and tannin, an astringent. Indian and Ceylon teas contain
more tannin than Chinese.

To process tea, the young shoots with their leaves and
buds are fermented briefly and then dried. About 2 per
cent of the world's production is unfermented, and the
leaves are boiled or steamed before being dried. The heat
inactivates ENZYMES that would otherwise turn them dark,
thus unfermented tea is green and fermented tea is black.
Oolong, exported mainly from Taiwan to the US, is partially fermented.

TENDERIZER

An ENZYME used to soften the flesh of older animals or
cheaper cuts of MEAT to make them more palatable. These
cuts contain the same NUTRIENTS as expensive steaks and
chops.

The earliest and still the most familiar tenderizer is
papain. It was isolated because Central American Indians
were known to rub meat with papaya or to wrap it in
papaya leaves before cooking it. The enzyme helps to break
down the gristle which consists of long, interconnected
PROTEINS called collagen. Bromelain from pineapples, ficin
from figs and enzymes from bacteria and fungi are also
now used.

In food PROCESSING, the tenderizer may be applied
directly to meat so as to break down the protein into
hydrolysates. Hydrolysates are AMINO ACIDS in solution
which can then be reconstituted as high-protein meat
substitutes. Tenderizers are also available from most shops
for domestic use. They are usually applied to the dish with
HERBS and spices shortly before cooking.

TENUATE ®

A SLIMMING AID available on prescription only. See APISATE for additional details.

TERONAC ®

A SLIMMING AID available on prescription only.

Teronac can cause constipation and insomnia, nervousness, headache, dizziness, skin rashes and temporary disturbances of urination and sexual potency. In a few patients, it may also disturb the heart slightly. It should never be used during pregnancy or breast feeding, nor should it be given to patients with peptic ULCERS, glaucoma, kidney, liver or heart disease or high blood pressure. Driving may be impaired after taking Teronac.

The common chemical name of the drug is mazindol. Though it is not chemically related to amphetamine, the earliest appetite suppressant, it is also an excitant and can create dependence.

TEXTURED VEGETABLE PROTEIN (TVP)

A MEAT substitute and ADDITIVE, also called novel PROTEIN and protein isolate.

SOYA BEANS are the principal source of TVP, but it may also be obtained from peanuts (groundnuts), oilseed, cottonseed, rape seed, coconut and sunflower. Oilseed protein may be cheaper and more widely available than soya.

TVP can be bought in many shops for home use. It comes either dry or canned as granules or lumps. Though TVP may be useful to extend mince or sausage meat, it cannot be said to taste like meat on its own. More finely milled TVP is used by food processors to create VEGETABLE 'chops' and even 'streaky bacon'. All such products must be labelled so the customer knows they contain TVP.

The substance is about 90 per cent protein and may also contain some IRON and B VITAMINS. However, TVP lacks an essential AMINO ACID, methionine, and should be supplemented with a small amount of animal protein or with YEAST.

Although it is a manufactured high-protein food, TVP should not be confused with meat hydrolysates. They are also high-protein foods (see TENDERIZER), but hydrolysates are derived from animal protein and contain all of the essential amino acids.

THICKENER

A food ADDITIVE also used as a STABILIZER. Thickeners increase the viscosity or thickness of a substance, for example, chocolate sauce for ice-cream or chocolate drinks. In home cookery, flour or cornflour are used as thickeners in making gravy, soups, etc. Domestic thickeners are less specific than commercial gums or STARCH derivatives such as amylose, and fulfil other roles: thus, flour is used to make BREAD.

Thickeners are also stabilizers, but not all stabilizers are used as thickeners. The stabilizers are designed to maintain a state, for example, the foam on a head of beer, or to prevent the release of liquid from gels as they age.

THYROID

1. A large endocrine gland in the lower neck and upper chest. 2. HORMONES properly called thyroxine and tri-iodothyroxine.

An endocrine gland is ductless; that is, it secretes chemicals, usually hormones, directly into the blood stream. The adrenal glands and the pituitary are also endocrine glands. The pancreas contains endocrine glands that make insulin and two other hormones (see CALCIUM, DIABETES) and it is also an exocrine gland secreting digestive ENZYMES through ducts into the intestine. The thyroid gland secretes thyroxine and tri-iodothyroxine directly into the blood. By means of these hormones, it helps to regulate growth and METABOLISM. In the blood and other tissues, the hormones ensure a more rapid turnover of AMINO ACIDS accompanied by greater ENERGY expenditure. Thus, the thyroid hormones also affect utilization of CARBOHYDRATE and FAT.

Needless to say, a thyroid pill for slimming has been attempted, but body chemistry is never so simple. The controls over hormone output are immensely complex. To tamper with a central regulatory mechanism in order to lose a few unfashionable pounds is foolhardy not to say dangerous. Fortunately, thyroid slimming pills are no longer available.

A diseased thyroid may produce either too little or too much thyroid hormone. Both malfunctions can cause weight gain. Treatment may involve IODINE, an element required for the synthesis of the thyroid hormones, drugs or surgery. Overweight due to thyroid malfunction is unusual, however, and it is a disease that only a doctor can treat.

TRACE ELEMENT
Gases or minerals required for health in amounts below one ten-thousandth of a gram (0.00001) in the adult body. They include copper, cobalt, FLUORINE, manganese, molybdenum, vanadium and zinc.

Like other NUTRIENTS, trace elements must be obtained from food. VEGETABLES are probably the best sources though fluorine, for example, may be taken from WATER.

Not all functions performed by trace elements are understood. Fluorine stabilizes tooth enamel but may also play a role in bone. Copper is required for a few ENZYMES to function and for the proper formation of red blood cells. Manganese may also be a necessary part of certain enzymes. Cobalt forms part of VITAMIN B_{12}.

TRIOSORBON ®
A dietary supplement and SLIMMING AID containing about 19 per cent PROTEIN including all of the essential AMINO ACIDS. FAT accounts for a further 19 per cent, and the balance is CARBOHYDRATE plus small quantities of VITAMINS and the most important MINERALS. According to the manufacturer, five 85g sachets per day meet normal adult nutritional needs.

Triosorbon is completely synthetic. As a food, it may be bought without a prescription. It is also used medically to feed patients with ABSORPTION diseases or as a tube feed when the patient cannot eat normally.

U

ULCERS

1. Any persistent break in the skin or a mucous membrane lining that fails to heal. 2. Specifically, a peptic ulcer which may be a gastric ulcer in the lining of the stomach or a duodenal ulcer in the lining of the duodenum, that portion of the small intestine nearest to the stomach.

There is no evidence that ulcers are connected with or caused by diet though the pain may be relieved by some food as well as by antacid drugs. In fact, the underlying causes of ulcers are unknown. They probably involve psychic as well as physiological factors.

The immediate trigger is the natural stomach ACID which prevents healing of a small break in the lining and attacks deeper layers of the stomach wall. Normally, stomach acid is produced only when there is food in the stomach. Tiny breaks in the mucous membrane occur constantly and are usually quickly replaced by new cells, but healing can be prevented by a malfunction in the production of acid or of pepsin, a digestive ENZYME.

Stomach acid production is regulated not only by the presence of food, however, but also by the main nervous connection to the brain, the vagus (see DIGESTIVE PROCESS). Even in the absence of food, the vagus nerve may stimulate both the activity of the stomach wall leading to lining damage and over-production of digestive juices. The vagal malfunction can be brought on by tension and either mental or physical stress. In effect, the stomach digests itself just like we digest tripe.

Antacids and special diets only relieve symptoms. Drugs may help the healing process, but rest is always essential. The rest must include the stomach wall itself and often requires tranquillizers. When the ulcer persists or new ones form, surgery may be tried either to remove the damaged part of the stomach or to cut the vagus nerve. Surgery is less common today, however, because doctors prefer new drugs which control symptoms and may allow the underlying malfunction to right itself.

Ulcers can be extremely dangerous. For example, bleeding into the abdominal cavity can lead to blood poisoning. On the other hand, there is no firm evidence that ulcers can become CANCER of the stomach or small intestine.

V

VAN ITALLIE CURE

An adaptation of the behaviourist slimming regimen (see WEIGHT WATCHERS). It is a non-commercial form of Weight Watchers and, therefore, much cheaper. The Van Itallie cure is recommended for a few like-minded overweight friends who want to set up a self-help group. No leader is necessary, and the group meets in the homes of its members.

Otherwise, the techniques are similar to other behavioural treatments. The slimmer must make a personal slimming contract and the commitment to continue with the group. Most important is the day-to-day maintenance of an eating record chart on which the slimmer notes the following points about every meal and snack:

1. Time taken for meal (the longer the better).
2. Place meal is eaten.
3. Physical position of eater; e.g., at table, armchair, etc.
4. Company or alone.
5. Associated activity; e.g., watching tv, listening to radio, conversation, scolding children.
6. Mood; e.g, bored, happy, rushed, tense.
7. Degree of hunger, if any.
8. Full description of meal or snack menu.
9. Total CALORIE intake.
10. Techniques used during meal to keep food intake

down, if any; e.g., no food on table apart from what is on plate, keeping food out of conversation, eating slowly.

This 'script' reinforces the slimming contract and provides the subject of discussion at the regular group meetings.

The labour involved in recording eating behaviour as well as the attention to detail is supposed to induce a contempt for food. There is also a practical consideration with psychological overtones: to record the details of every meal and snack consumes precious time. Fancy dishes take more time to record than simple dishes which may mean that Calorie-packed sauces, for example, will gradually play a smaller role in the diet.

The Van Itallie slimmer also learns that if he or she is to lose weight, Calorie intake must be over-balanced by Calorie expenditure. There are no set diet programmes but EXERCISE and awareness of the ENERGY required by certain activities is a part of the cure.

VEGAN
A person who eats only plant foods and excludes all animal products from the diet including butter, CHEESE, EGGS and MILK.

The vegan diet originated in poor regions such as southern India where hardship led to the evolution of elaborate mystical explanations intended to reduce both apathy and resistance among those people, often the producers of what food there was, who were forced to accept the regimen. In the more affluent western world, many people become vegans because they see no real distinction between killing animals for their flesh and expropriating animal products produced for the health and maintenance of the animal population. It is also argued that the vegan diet is more healthful. Vegans recognize that animal products contain saturated FATS which may be associated with a greater risk of heart disease and high blood pressure.

A diet without animal products can provide all NUTRIENTS with two exceptions: the essential AMINO ACID, methionine, and VITAMIN B_{12}. It should be borne in mind that methionine is essential because under normal circumstances the body does not synthesize enough to meet its needs. We do make some, and it is possible that the healthy body will adapt to a relative shortage. Healthy people living relatively sedentary lives may get by. After injury, during illness or pregnancy, after bouts of hard physical EXERCISE and during growth, however, the committed vegan would be wise to add YEAST to his or her diet, though yeast is a fungus, or to eat a synthetic food supplement such as COMPLAN to which the essential nutrients have been added. The absence of vitamin B_{12} is more serious. A few plants contain small amounts (see COMFREY), but supplements should be taken, especially by children and pregnant and nursing women.

The improved health and sense of well-being that vegans feel is often associated with the less stressful life-style that many adopt. In the west, they are usually people who opt out of the rat race and accept much lower living standards. Information about a vegan diet can be obtained from The Vegan Society, 47 Highlands Road, Leatherhead, Surrey.

VEGETABLE

1. Any plant food that is not a FRUIT or NUT. 2. In common use, a vegetable is a legume, a root or a leaf. (See also CEREAL, PULSE.)

The legumes include all kinds of peas as well as SOYA BEANS and other pulses. They contain PROTEINS and FAT. Amounts vary with the species. Ordinary peas, runner beans, kidney beans and baked beans are about 17 per cent protein and 1 per cent OIL. The protein is of limited quality because it lacks one or more essential AMINO ACID. The legumes are good sources of FIBRE, MINERALS and the B VITAMINS and vitamin C. It is also true, however, that legumes tend to cause flatulence. Some of the less common beans, like butter beans, contain toxic substances which must be destroyed by soaking and boiling before eating. For example, kidney beans should be fast-boiled for at least 10 minutes before they are used. On the other hand, peas and runner beans may be eaten raw with perfect safety and possibly some additional fibre and B vitamins.

The roots include potatoes, carrots, beets, parsnips, turnips, yams, sweet potatoes, Jerusalem artichokes and TAPIOCA or cassava. They contain useful quantities of digestible CARBOHYDRATE in the form of STARCH, minerals and vitamins, especially vitamins A and C.

Leaf vegetables have little protein and even less digestible carbohydrate and fat. They are good sources of fibre, minerals and vitamins, especially vitamin C. The largest family are the brassicas which include cabbage, cauliflower, brussels sprouts, broccoli and globe artichokes. A second major family is spinach and related vegetables such as rhubarb. Unless the leaf vegetables are cooked while they are still fresh, the loss of vitamin C is considerable. Refrigeration delays vitamin loss. Frozen vegetables should be cooked from the frozen state to preserve vitamin C, but heat, the presence of oxygen or of BASES also destroys this vitamin.

B vitamins may be leached out of vegetables during cooking, but some may be recovered if the WATER is used as stock. All vegetables lose vitamins during storage and preparation such as scraping or chopping.

Vegetables such as spinach contain oxalic acid (see CAL-CIUM, IRON). Minerals are poorly absorbed (see ABSORPTION) in the presence of this substance.

Uncooked vegetables have very little more fibre than the same vegetable cooked. Fibre consists of CELLULOSE and other indigestible carbohydrates which are softened but not removed by cooking. On the other hand, over-cooking should always be avoided. It destroys vitamins, as noted above, and reduces taste. Vegetables should be served *al dente*, just chewable like good pasta. SALT and fat-based sauces add nutrients and sometimes taste to vegetables, but they also create dietary problems. Sauces add CALORIES to dishes that otherwise have very few, and salt can increase water retention which can increase both weight and blood pressure. As a meal, vegetables are like dairy products: they can often stand on their own.

VEGETARIAN

A person who eats only plant foods, dairy products and EGGS.

In the west, vegetarianism is based on several considerations: a dislike for FISH and MEAT, compassion for animals, environmental arguments and the health arguments – the relative infrequency of heart and circulatory diseases and CANCER in the third world where people tend to be vegetarians. In the third world, vegetarianism is often a matter of necessity. People are too poor to buy a nourishing variety of vegetables such as high-protein PULSES, let alone dairy products or EGGS, even if the existing distribution system made them available. They frequently suffer from protein-deficiency diseases (see KWASHIORKOR), and less commonly die of cancer or heart disease in part because they die from other causes. Their life-expectancy at birth is still as much as thirty years less than it is in the west where the familiar causes of death tend to be diseases of older people. For the environmental and economic arguments in favour of vegetarianism, see MEAT.

A vegetarian diet can be just as well-balanced as one containing meat. Dairy products and eggs are animal foods, of course, and provide the essential NUTRIENTS, the AMINO ACIDS and VITAMIN B_{12}, which a VEGAN diet lacks.

VERY LOW CALORIE DIET (VLCD)

A food intake that supplies less than 500 CALORIES per day. The food may be entirely liquid. Such an extreme diet can only be justified by life-threatening OBESITY and must never be undertaken without a doctor's advice. However, there is an exception that points a moral: famine relief organizations now make available a wheat-flour-based biscuit which can be manufactured and transported very cheaply. Four biscuits will sustain life but supply just 500 Calories.

Men on VLCDs can expect to lose 4 to 10lb a week, and women, 3 to 5lb. In 1977, liquid diets were the sole or principal source of food for almost 100,000 American women who were undergoing self-imposed weight-loss diets. However, the widespread use of VLCDs stopped abruptly when they were associated with sudden deaths among otherwise healthy people. Fifty-eight deaths were reported in the United States among VLCD users, of which seventeen were due to serious heart abnormality. No exact cause has been assigned to the abnormality, but it is possible that the low-calorie intake administered a physical and psychological shock severe enough to stress the body unduly. It is interesting that the more obese the dieter, the less he or she risks sudden death.

Currently available commercial VLCD products are well balanced nutritionally (see LIMMITS, SLENDER). The problem with their use, apart from the serious risk from shock, is that most people find it very hard to maintain their new body weight once they stop using VLCDs. Every dieter knows it is not easy to hold on to the losses, as it were, and the problem is often worse for the obese, especially if they are compulsive eaters.

VINEGAR

A condiment containing acetic ACID made by fermenting barley (malt vinegar), grape juice or WINE (wine vinegar), cider or SPIRITS. Vinegar contains almost no CALORIES and makes a useful salad dressing for slimming diets. It cannot be said to cause weight loss, though.

Acetic acid is a PRESERVATIVE. Vinegar contains not less than 4 per cent but may have much more. Commercial vinegar also contains COLOUR, usually caramel, and it may have another preservative, sulphur dioxide. Most vinegar contains traces of MINERALS and B VITAMINS from the original ferment.

VITAMIN

A NUTRIENT, very small amounts of which must be obtained from the daily diet to maintain life. The word, 'vitamin', originally spelled vitamine, was invented by a German chemist, Funk, who identified the first vitamin in 1911. The word means amine of life.

The ultimate effect of any vitamin deficiency that persists is death. However, each vitamin plays a distinctive role in METABOLISM. Long before death, therefore, its absence causes characteristic symptoms and diseases.

The table on pages 200–201 lists the known vitamins, their common chemical names, their best food sources, although there may be many others, the major physiological jobs they do (again, there may be others), the most obvious early symptoms of vitamin deficiency and a few useful remarks.

Although from time to time reports identify other chemicals as vitamins, there is no proof that they fit the definition given above.

The average western diet contains adequate amounts of all vitamins. Supplements may be needed during pregnancy, but your doctor will tell you if they are required. Supplements may also be prescribed after a debilitating illness when the patient has been unable to eat. For most people, however, vitamin pills and preparations are expensive but valueless gimmicks. Indeed, with vitamin A caution is needed because it is possible to die of a surfeit. Vitamin A is held in the body by FAT and is not quickly excreted. Although poisoning by vitamins D, E and K have never been reported, it is theoretically possible for the same reasons. As to the claim that vitamin C in large doses prevents or cures the common cold, there is unfortunately no experimental support for it. Vitamin C can probably do no harm, but by and large, you will save both time and money if you ask your doctor before buying any vitamin supplement.

W

WATER
H_2O. Water is quite as essential for life as any NUTRIENT. In the climate of the UK and the US, the average adult needs about a pint and a half of water every day to replace losses through sweating and urination. In hot climates

Vitamin	Common chemical name	Best food sources	Major physiological roles	Symptoms of deficiency	Remarks
A	Retinol	Carrots, liver, eggs	Sight, skin health	Night blindness, eye disease, skin disease, nervous disorders	It is possible to be poisoned by too much vitamin A
B_1	Thiamine	Liver, bread, milk	Transformation of carbohydrate to energy	Beriberi: weakness, nervous disorders	All B vitamins: it is not possible to eat too much, but no advantages accrue from excesses
B_2	Riboflavin	As B_1	As B_1	Eye damage, weakness, inflammation of mucous membranes	Deficiency usually accompanies deficiency of B_3
B_3, Niacin	Nicotinic acid	As B_1	As B_1	Pellagra: weakness, eye damage, dementia	See B_2
B_6	Pyridoxine	As B_1	Protein metabolism	Skin damage, anaemia, convulsions	
B_{12}	Cyanocobalamin	Animal products, especially offal	Formation of blood cells, coatings of many nerves	Anaemia, severe nervous disorders	Absorption requires intrinsic factor (see DIGESTIVE PROCESS)
Folic acid	Pteroylmono-glutamic acid	As B_1	Formation of blood cells	Anaemia	
Biotin	Biotin	As B_1 but most food	As B_1	Nervous disorders, weakness. In infants: acid-base imbalance	Deficiency is rare. Possible causes: genetic, excess egg white

C	Ascorbic acid	Citrus fruit, dark green vegetables	Carbohydrate metabolism, energy formation, protein formation	Scurvy: weakness, haemorrhage	
D	Calciferol	Fatty fish, fish liver oils	Utilization of calcium and potassium	Rickets. In adults: osteomalacia	Also derived from sunshine on skin. Deficiencies seen in Britain especially among Indians and Pakistanis who obtain little from customary diet and have too little sunshine
E	Tocopherol	All foods, vegetable oils	Formation of blood cells	Anaemia	Deficiency is rare. No evidence that it protects against heart disease
K	Phytonadione, Menadione	All foods, but human source is probably intestinal bacteria	Formation of factors that permit blood clotting	Bleeding	Deficiency is rare

during periods of intensive EXERCISE or hard work, much more water is needed accompanied by SALT. Depending on the climate and the health of the person, it is possible to survive without water for about four days. Gradually, the body fluids become too depleted to support life.

Drowning, on the other hand, occurs when the victim takes in water rather than air through the lungs. Because water can pass through the membranes in the lungs like air, the blood becomes too dilute very quickly, and water pours into the tissues under osmotic pressure. Air is also excluded, of course, but death is usually caused by flooding rather than strangulation.

It is fatal to drink salt water because the salt build-up in the body is too much for the kidneys to handle unless they simultaneously excrete more water than the body contains. In other words, salt water can cause fatal dehydration.

Yet despite these crisis conditions, the need for water is compelling. The sensation of thirst is triggered by yet another delicate physiological balance, brain cells that measure the quantity of body fluids against current chemical and physical needs. Indeed, its physical and chemical complexities make water a subject of delight to the intellectually thirsty too because, as has been said before, if it didn't already exist, someone would have had to invent it.

One final interesting fact about the relation between water and health: hard water is associated with a lower risk from heart disease. It is not known whether this is because minerals in hard water are somehow protective, or because in soft water some harmful factor is unmasked.

WEIGHT WATCHERS Ⓡ

One of the first commercial uses of behavioural techniques combined with a slimming diet to achieve weight loss.

Behavioural therapy is based on the theory that we learn habits as well as information by a series of repeated responses to stimuli. If the stimulus is noxious like a bad taste, we avoid it. In the process, we learn to avoid the substance that tastes bad. If the stimulus is pleasant like a sweet taste, we learn to accept it and to anticipate the source of the stimulus. We also try to increase the pleasant stimuli, for example by eating things that we have learned taste good or look as though they might.

Unfortunately, food that tastes good may also make us FAT. Fat is or ought to be a noxious stimulus. The trouble is that for overweight and obese people, the pattern of their food responses is too powerful to be easily modified by the intellectual realization that overweight is unhealthy. Behaviour therapy for slimming is designed to modify learned food responses by replacing them with new ones.

According to the theory, new responses will be learned only if the stimuli are pleasant, and if the old stimuli can be made unpleasant. Thus, weight loss is a positively-pleasant stimulus. Disapproval because of failure to lose weight, especially the disapproval of other people in the same boat, is a powerful disincentive to over-eating. Behavioural therapy can take different forms, but there is statistical evidence that combined with a slimming diet, it produces a permanent weight loss in more people than either behavioural therapy or a slimming diet alone.

Weight Watchers begins by inviting the would-be weight loser to attend a weekly class led by a lecturer. In a class, other people are present from the outset. You are not having to cope alone. Membership in the class requires payment of a registration fee and a fee for each class. In the UK, weight watchers do not sign a contract to attend a certain number of classes as they do in the US. They know, however, that the course consists of sixteen weekly classes. If they drop out, they can rejoin on payment of a new registration fee. Fees are also powerful stimuli to get value for money.

With the lecturer, the new member works out a goal weight. He or she is then given diet suggestions and recommendations all of which recognize that 1. the fewer CALORIES you eat, the more quickly you will lose weight, and 2. a balanced diet is necessary for health. No diet is mandatory.

The member is asked to keep a food diary. For each meal and snack, the member is to write down the time, duration, type and amount of food eaten, degree of hunger before eating, mood, eating place (armchair, table, etc.) and position (straight, reclining, etc.) and other people present. These diaries are to be brought to class where they form the basis for a discussion and comparison with the diaries kept by the other class members. In addition, the lecturer weighs each member each week and maintains a weight record which is open for the others to see.

These group activities and the food diary are believed to be as important as the slimming diet for achieving weight loss. Above all, slimmers are expected to learn to maintain their new body weights because they have built up new habits that enable them to eat fewer calories if not less food. Weight Watchers give an incentive for weight maintenance by asking members who have successfully achieved their goal weight during a course to attend later classes at no charge.

See also VAN ITALLIE CURE.

WHO
World Health Organization. A United Nations body with headquarters in Geneva. With the cooperation and approval of member nations, it sets standards, for example, for acceptable food ADDITIVES, recommends public health measures, provides expert advice and assistance and conducts or sponsors research on health and disease both in the field and in laboratories throughout the world. Its clients are nations rather than institutions, and the principal thrust of WHO activities is directed toward the neediest nations in the third world.

WHOLEFOOD
A promotional word implying that nothing has been added and nothing removed. Other than EGGS, it is not easy to think of a food that has had nothing added to it or removed from it before eating. Even eggs have lost their shells. Perhaps a few NUTS, although the shells are usually waste, and salad foods like lettuce, tomatoes and CUCUMBERS also fit the description.

Most vegetables are cooked and will lose NUTRIENTS even if they were freshly picked. Wholemeal BREAD contains ADDITIVES unless it is homemade. We usually throw away the rind, core and seeds of FRUIT. In short, the word 'wholefood' may increase the price of the product but not the information about it.

See also HEALTH FOOD.

WINE

1. The ferment of grape juice. 2. Ferments of other VEGETABLES, FRUITS and flowers; i.e., country wines.

The ALCOHOL content of country wines is variable but rarely higher than 4 per cent. Table wines contain less than 12 per cent. FERMENTATION is stopped when this level is reached. In dry wines, the SUGAR will have been almost entirely converted to alcohol. Conversely, sweet wines still contain some of the fruit sugar. CALORIES in both come largely from the alcohol, however. The COLOURS and FLAVOURS of wines depend primarily on the grapes used, but the presence of contaminants during fermentation also plays a role. Wines may contain naturally-occurring tannins, ACIDS, gums and pectins. Sulphur dioxide is a permitted PRESERVATIVE.

The designation, *appellation controlé*, means that the label tells the truth about the source of the wine and where it was bottled. If it is called Beaune, it must have been fermented from grapes grown near that French town, but unless the label says otherwise, it need not have been bottled there. English wine means that the grapes were grown in England. British wine, on the other hand, is made from grapes grown abroad but fermented and bottled here.

Sparkling wine including 'champagne' is made by adding a little sugar and YEAST to a bottled wine. After six to eight weeks at a constant temperature of 16° to 19°C, the cork and yeast are removed, usually by freezing the bottle neck and pulling out the cork with the yeast which has become attached to it. A new cork is then wired into the bottle.

The fortified wines, sherry, port, madeira, marsala and

vermouth, have alcohol added to the original ferment so that they contain up to 17 per cent alcohol. Bitter flavours and sugars are also added to vermouth.

All wines contain some MINERALS and B VITAMINS. In respect to these constituents, red and white wine do not vary significantly.

Y

YEAST
A family of fungi that live and multiply by converting SUGAR to ALCOHOL and carbon dioxide. They have great commercial value for baking, brewing and wine-making. In baking, heat drives off the alcohol, but the carbon dioxide causes the dough to rise.

The yeasts are also good sources of MINERALS, PROTEIN and the B VITAMINS. The protein is of high quality because it supplies all essential AMINO ACIDS. They are often used today as a source of synthetic or novel protein (see TEXTURED VEGETABLE PROTEIN). Dried yeast may be eaten as a supplement and is especially suitable for VEGANS. Some people find its taste unpleasant, but the taste can be disguised by sprinkling it on other food.

There are three major types of yeast used commercially: bakers' yeast, brewers' yeast and torula yeast. They differ in their speed of action and rate of growth, and there are moderate variations in their NUTRIENT content.

YOGA
Yoga seeks perfect mental and physical health to remove bodily functions and problems as barriers to the achievement of peace and insight. Food and diet are thus adjuncts of this achievement. Indeed, enjoyment of food is in a sense contradictory to the goal. To those who can commit themselves to the purposes behind the practice of yoga, therefore, its techniques may well be useful as a means of appetite control.

Yoga is from a Sanskrit word which is also the origin of

the word yoke. In Hindu religious philosophy, the yoke is the Union of man with a Supreme Being. In common use, yoga means meditation, mental concentration and ascetic practices which are used to attain this union. The many branches or schools of yoga emphasize different aspects of these three techniques, but all of them prescribe certain postures (*asanas*) and breathing methods (*pranayama*).

YOGHURT

A MILK product made by bacteria which convert the milk SUGAR to lactic acid partially curdling the milk. Lactic acid suppresses harmful bacteria and acts as a PRESERVATIVE. Yoghurt can be kept in the refrigerator for about two weeks, and it can also be frozen.

The NUTRIENTS in plain yoghurt are about the same as in whole boiled milk. Fat-free and low-fat yoghurt is made from skimmed milk or skim milk powder. FRUIT yoghurts have added fruit and sugar. They can easily be made at home by adding fruit or jam to plain yoghurt.

Two bacteria are commonly used to manufacture yoghurt, *Lactobacillus bulgaricus* and *Streptococcus thermophilus*, because they help each other to grow. Commercial plain yoghurt can be used as a culture to start homemade yoghurt, but the milk to which it is added must be boiled even though it is also both pasteurized and fresh. Otherwise, in the warm conditions required for the culture to grow, harmful bacteria in the whole milk will multiply before enough lactic acid has accumulated to inhibit them. The milk will go sour.

Many variants on yoghurt are eaten. Kumiss, usually made from goat's or yak's milk, contains YEASTS which produce ALCOHOL in addition to the yoghurt bacilli that produce lactic acid. Acidophilus milk is yoghurt made with *Lactobacillus acidophilus*, a bacterium normally found in the human bowel. Acidophilus milk is used to check diarrhoea caused by antibiotics that kill intestinal bacteria.

Appendix I. Recommended Daily Intakes of Energy and Nutrients by Age, Sex and Status*

Age	Energy kilo-calories	Energy mega-joules	Protein grams	B vitamins Thiamine milligrams	Riboflavin milligrams	Nicotinic acid milligram equivalents	Vitamin C milligrams	Vitamin A microgram equivalents	Vitamin D micrograms	Calcium milligrams	Iron milligrams
Boys and Girls											
Up to 12 months	800	3.3	20	0.3	0.4	5	15	450	10	600	6
1 year	1200	5.0	30	0.5	0.6	7	20	300	10	500	7
2 years	1400	5.9	35	0.6	0.7	8	20	300	10	500	7
3 to 4 years	1600	6.7	40	0.6	0.8	9	20	300	10	500	8
5 to 6 years	1800	7.5	45	0.7	0.9	10	20	300	2.5	500	8
7 to 8 years	2100	8.8	53	0.8	1.0	11	20	400	2.5	500	10
Boys											
9 to 11 years	2500	10.5	63	1.0	1.2	14	25	575	2.5	700	13
12 to 14 years	2800	11.7	70	1.1	1.4	16	25	725	2.5	700	14
15 to 17 years	3000	12.6	75	1.2	1.7	19	30	750	2.5	600	15
Girls											
9 to 11 years	2300	9.6	58	0.9	1.2	13	25	575	2.5	700	13
12 to 14 years	2300	9.6	58	0.9	1.4	16	25	725	2.5	700	14
15 to 17 years	2300	9.6	58	0.9	1.4	16	30	750	2.5	600	15

Men

18 to 34 years sedentary	2700	11.3	68	1.1	1.7	18	30	750	2.5	500	10
moderately active	3000	12.6	75	1.2	1.7	18	30	750	2.5	500	10
very active	3600	15.1	90	1.4	1.7	18	30	750	2.5	500	10
35 to 64 years sedentary	2600	10.9	65	1.0	1.7	18	30	750	2.5	500	10
moderately active	2900	12.1	73	1.2	1.8	18	30	750	2.5	500	10
very active	3600	15.1	90	1.4	1.7	18	30	750	2.5	500	10
65 to 74 years sedentary life	2350	9.8	59	0.9	1.7	18	30	750	2.5	500	10
75 and over sedentary life	2100	8.8	53	0.8	1.7	18	30	750	2.5	500	10
Women											
18 to 54 years most occupations	2200	9.2	55	0.9	1.3	15	30	750	2.5	500	12
55 to 74 years sedentary life	2050	8.6	51	0.8	1.3	15	30	750	2.5	500	10
75 and over sedentary life	1900	8.0	48	0.7	1.3	15	30	750	2.5	500	10
Pregnancy, 3 to 9 months	2400	10.0	60	1.0	1.6	18	60	750	10†	1200**	15
Breast feeding	2700	11.3	68	1.1	1.8	21	60	1200	10	1200	15

* Based on Recommended Intakes of Nutrients for the United Kingdom DHSS Rep. Pub. Health & Med. Sub. no. 120 1969
† for all 9 months
** last 3 months

Appendix II. 'E' Numbers

List of food additives to which 'E' numbers have been allocated by the European Economic Community. NB: this is not a comprehensive list of additives permitted for use in food in the United Kingdom. For key to letter symbols (e.g., TN), see end of list.

'E' Number	Substance	UK (i.e. England and Wales) Regulations
100	Curcumin	C
TN 101a	Riboflavin-5'-phosphate	C
101	Riboflavin (Lactoflavin)	C
102	Tartrazine	C
104	Quinoline Yellow	C
TN 107	Yellow 2G	C
110	Sunset Yellow FCF (Orange Yellows S)	C
120	Cochineal (Carmine of cochineal or Carminic acid)	C
122	Carmoisine (Azorubine)	C
123	Amaranth	C
124	Ponceau 4R (Cochineal Red A)	C
127	Erythrosine BS	C
TN 128	Red 2G	C
131	Patent Blue V	C
132	Indigo Carmine (Indigotine)	C
TN 133	Brilliant Blue FCF	C
140	Chlorophyll	C
141	Copper complexes of chlorophyll and chlorophyllins	C
142	Green S (Acid Brilliant Green BS or Lissamine Green)	C

'E' Number	Substance	UK (i.e. England and Wales) Regulations
150	Caramel	C
151	Black PN (Brilliant Black BN)	C
153	Carbon Black (Vegetable Carbon)	C
TN 154	Brown FK	C
TN 155	Chocolate Brown HT	C
160(a)	alpha-carotene, beta-carotene, gamma-carotene	C
160(b)	Annatto, bixin, norbixin	C
160(c)	Capsanthin (Capsorubin)	C
160(d)	Lycopene	C
160(e)	beta-Apo-8'-carotenal (C_{30})	C
160(f)	Ethyl ester of beta-apo-8'-carotenoic acid (C_{30})	C
161(a)	Flavoxanthin	C
161(b)	Lutein	C
161(c)	Cryptoxanthin	C
161(d)	Rubixanthin	C
161(e)	Violaxanthin	C
161(f)	Rhodoxanthin	C
161(g)	Canthaxanthin	C
162	Beetroot Red (Betanin)	C
163	Anthocyanins	C
170	Calcium carbonate	M
171	Titanium dioxide	C
172	Iron oxides and hydroxides	C
173	Aluminium	C
174	Silver	C
175	Gold	C
180	Pigment Rubine (Lithol Rubine BK)	C
200	Sorbic acid	P
201	Sodium sorbate	P
202	Potassium sorbate	P
203	Calcium sorbate	P
210	Benzoic acid	P
211	Sodium benzoate	P
212	Potassium benzoate	P
213	Calcium benzoate	P

'E' Number	Substance	UK (i.e. England and Wales) Regulations
214	Ethyl 4-hydroxybenzoate (Ethyl para-hydroxybenzoate)	P
215	Ethyl 4-hydroxybenzoate, sodium salt (Sodium ethyl *para*-hydroxybenzoate)	P
216	Propyl 4-hydroxybenzoate (Propyl *para*-hydroxybenzoate)	P
217	Propyl 4-hydroxybenzoate, sodium salt (Sodium propyl *para*-hydroxybenzoate)	P
218	Methyl 4-hydroxybenzoate (Methyl para-hydroxybenzoate)	P
219	Methyl 4-hydroxybenzoate, sodium salt (Sodium methyl para-hydroxybenzoate)	P
220	Sulphur dioxide	P
221	Sodium sulphite	P
222	Sodium hydrogen sulphite (Sodium bisulphite)	P
223	Sodium metabisulphite	P
224	Potassium metabisulphite	P
226	Calcium sulphite	P
227	Calcium hydrogen sulphite (Calcium bisulphite)	P
230	Biphenyl (Diphenyl)	P
231	2-Hydroxybiphenyl (orthophenylphenyl)	
232	Sodium biphenyl-2-yl oxide (Sodium orthophenylphenate)	P
233	2-(Thiazol-4 yl) benzimidazole (Thiabendazole)	P
TN 234	Nisin	P
239	Hexamine (Hexamethyl enetetramine)	P
249	Potessium nitrite	P
250	Sodium nitrate	P

'E' Number	Substance	UK (i.e. England and Wales) Regulations
251	Sodium nitrate	P
252	Potassium nitrate	P
260	Acetic acid	M
261	Potassium acetate	M
262	Sodium hydrogen diacetate	M
TN 262	Sodium acetate	M
263	Calcium acetate	M
270	Lactic acid	M
280	Propionic acid	P
281	Sodium propionate	P
282	Calcium propionate	P
283	Potassium propionate	P
290	Carbon dioxide	M
TN 296	Malic acid	M
TN 297	Fumaric acid	M
300	L-Ascorbic acid	A
301	Sodium-L-ascorbate	A
302	Calcium-L-ascorbate	A
304	6-O-Palmitoyl-L-ascorbic acid (Ascorbyl palmitate)	A
306	Extracts of natural origin rich in tocopherols	A
307	Synthetic *alpha*-tocopherol	A
308	Synthetic *gamma*-tocopherol	A
309	Synthetic *delta*-tocopherol	A
310	Propyl gallate	A
311	Octyl gallate	A
312	Dodecyl gallate	A
320	Butylated hydroxyanisole (BHA)	A
321	Butylated hydroxytoluene (BHT)	A
322	Lecithins	E
325	Sodium lactate	M
326	Potassium lactate	M
327	Calcium lactate	M
330	Citric acid	M
331	Sodium dihydrogen citrate (*mono*Sodium citrate)	M
	*di*Sodium citrate	M
	*tri*Sodium citrate	M

'E' Number	Substance	UK (i.e. England and Wales) Regulations
332	Potassium dihydrogen citrate (*mono*Potassium citrate)	M
	*tri*Potassium citrate	M
333	*mono*Calcium citrate	M
	*di*Calcium citrate	M
	*tri*Calcium citrate	M
334	L-(+)-Tartaric acid	M
335	*mono*Sodium L-(+)-tartrate	M
	*di*Sodium L-(+)-tartrate	
336	*mono*Potassium L-(+)-tartrate (Cream of tartar)	M
	*di*Potassium L-(+)-tartrate	M
337	Potassium sodium L-(+)-tartrate	M
338	Orthophosphoric acid (Phosphoric acid)	M
339	Sodium dihydrogen orthophosphate	M
	*di*Sodium hydrogen orthophosphate	M
	*tri*Sodium orthophosphate	M
340	Potassium dihydrogen orthophosphate	M
	*di*Potassium hydrogen orthophosphate	M
	*tri*Potassium orthophosate	M
341	Calcium tetrahydrogen diorthophosphate	M
	Calcium hydrogen orthophosphate	M
	*tri*Calcium diorthophosphate	M
TN 350	Sodium malate	M
	Sodium hydrogen malate	M
TN 351	Potassium malate	M
TN 352	Calcium malate	M
	Calcium hydrogen malate	M
TN 353	Metatartaric acid	M
TN 355	Adipic acid	M
TN 363	Succinic acid	M
TN 370	1,-4-Heptono-lactone	M

'E' Number	Substance	UK (i.e. England and Wales) Regulations
TN 375	Nicotinic acid	M
TN 380	*Tri*-ammonium citrate	M
TN 381	Ammonium ferric citrate	M
TN 385	Calcium *di*sodium EDTA (calcium disodium ethylenediamine – NNN 'N' tetra – acetate)	M
400	Alginic acid	E
401	Sodium alginate	E
402	Potassium alginate	E
403	Ammonium alginate	E
404	Calcium alginate	E
405	Propane-1,2-diol alginate (Propylene glycol alginate)	E
406	Agar	E
407	Carrageenan	E
410	Locust bean gum (Carob gum)	E
412	Guar gum	E
413	Tragacanth	E
414	Gum arabic (Acacia)	E
415	Xanthan Gum	E
TN 416	Karaya Gum	E
420	Sorbitol	SW
	Sorbitol syrup	SW
421	Mannitol	SW
422	Glycerol	S
440(a)	Pectin	E
440(b)	Amidated pectin	E
TN 442	Ammonium phosphatides	E
450(a)	*di*Sodium dihydrogen diphosphate	M
	*tri*Sodium diphosphate	M
	*tetra*Sodium diphosphate	M
	*tetra*Potassium diphosphate	M
450(b)	*penta*Sodium triphosphate	M
	*penta*Potassium triphosphate	M
450(c)	Sodium polyphosphates	M
	Potassium polyphosphates	M
460	Microcrystalline cellulose	E
	Alpha-cellulose (Powdered cellulose)	M

'E' Number	Substance	UK (i.e. England and Wales) Regulations
461	Methylcellulose	E
463	Hydroxypropylcellulose	E
464	Hydroxypropylmethylcellulose	E
465	Ethylmethylcellulose	E
466	Carboxymethylcellulose, sodium salt (CMC)	E
470	Sodium, potassium and calcium salts of fatty acids	E
471	Mono- and di-glycerides of fatty acids	E
472(a)	Acetic acid esters of mono- and di-glycerides of fatty acids	E
472(b)	Lactic acid esters of mono- and di-glycerides of fatty acids (Lactoglycerides)	E
472(c)	Citric acid esters of mono- and di-glycerides of fatty acids (Citroglycerides)	E
472(e)	Mono- and Diacetyltartaric acid esters of mono- and di-glycerides of fatty acids	E
473	Sucrose esters of fatty acids	E
474	Sucroglycerides	E
475	Polyglycerol esters of fatty acids	E
TN 476	Polyglycerol polyricinoleate	E
477	Propane-1,2-diol esters of fatty acids	E
TN 478	Lactylated fatty acid esters of glycerol and propane-1,2-diol	E
481	Sodium stearoyl-2-lactylate	E
482	Calcium stearoyl-2-lactylate	E
483	Stearyl tartrate	E

All of the following are Temporary Numbers (TN):

| 491 | Sorbitan monostearate | E |
| 492 | Sorbitan tristearate | E |

'E' Number	Substance	UK (i.e. England and Wales) Regulations
493	Sorbitan monolaurate	E
494	Sorbitan mono-oleate	E
495	Sorbitan monopalmitate	E
572	Magnesium monopalmitate	M
500	Sodium carbonate	M
	Sodium hydrogen carbonate (Bicarbonate of soda)	M
	Sodium sesquicarbonate	M
501	Potassium carbonate	M
	Potassium hydrogen carbonate	M
503	Ammonium carbonate	M
	Ammonium hydrogen carbonate	M
504	Magnesium carbonate, heavy	M
	Magnesium carbonate, light	M
507	Hydrochloric acid	M
508	Potassium chloride	M
509	Calcium chloride	M
	Calcium chloride anhydrous	M
510	Ammonium chloride	M
513	Sulphuric acid	M
514	Sodium sulphate	M
515	Potassium sulphate	M
516	Calcium sulphate	M
518	Magnesium sulphate	M
524	Sodium hydroxide	M
525	Potassium hydroxide	M
526	Calcium hydroxide	M
527	Ammonium hydroxide	M
528	Magnesium hydroxide	M
529	Calcium oxide	M
530	Magnesium oxide, heavy	M
	Magnesium oxide, light	M
535	Sodium ferrocyanide (sodium hexacyanoferrate II)	M
536	Potassium ferrocyanide (potassium hexacyanoferrate II)	M
540	diCalcium diphosphate	M

'E' Number	Substance	UK (i.e. England and Wales) Regulations
541	Sodium aluminium phosphate acidic	M
	Sodium aluminium phosphate basic	M
542	Edible bone phosphate	M
544	Calcium polyphosphates	M
545	Ammonium polyphosphates	M
551	Silicon *di*oxide (silica)	M
552	Calcium silicate	M
553(a)	Magnesium silicate, synthetic	M
	Magnesium *tri*silicate	M
553(b)	Talc	M
554	Sodium aluminium silicate	M
556	Calcium aluminium silicate	M
558	Bentonite	M
559	Kaolin, light	M
	Kaolin, heavy	M
575	Glucono-*delta*-lactone (D-Glucono-1,5-lactone)	M
576	Sodium gluconate	M
577	Potassium gluconate	M
578	Calcium gluconate	M
620	L-Glutamic Acid ø	M
621	*Mono*sodium glutamate or MSG (Sodium hydrogen L-glutamate)	M
622	*Mono*potassium glutamate ø (Potassium hydrogen L-glutamate	M
623	Calcium glutamate ø (Calcium *di*hydrogen *di*-L-glutamate)	M
627	Sodium guanylate (Guanosine 5'-[*di*sodium phosphate])	M
631	Sodium inosinate (Inosine 5'-[*di*sodium phosphate])	M
635	Sodium 5'-ribonucleotide	M
900	Dimethylpolysiloxane	M
901	Beeswax, white	M
	Beeswax, yellow	M
903	Carnauba wax	M

'E' Number	Substance	UK (i.e. England and Wales) Regulations
904	Shellac	M
920	L-cysteine hydrochloride (anhydrous and monohydrate)	Bread and Flour
924	Potassium bromate	Bread and Flour
925	Chlorine	Bread and Flour
926	Chlorine dioxide	Bread and Flour
927	Azoformamide (azodicarbonide)	Bread and Flour

Key

A = Antioxidants

C = Colours

E = Emulsifiers and Stabilizers

M = Miscellaneous Additives. Classes are: acids, anticaking and antifoaming agents, bases, buffers, firming and glazing agents, humefactants, liquid freezants, packaging gases, propellants, release agents, sequestrants, bulking aids and flavour modifiers. Some additives fall into more than one class.

P = Preservatives

S = Solvents

SW = Sweeteners

TN = Temporary Number. These have been allocated by the EEC and may be used when they have been incorporated into UK law in place of the specific name of the additive.